anything
but silent

our family's journey through
childhood apraxia of speech

anything but silent

our family's journey through childhood apraxia of speech

kathy & kate hennessy

WORD ASSOCIATION PUBLISHERS
www.wordassociation.com
1.800.827.7903

ISBN: 978-1-59571-879-2

Library of Congress Control Number: 2013906043

Designed and published by
Word Association Publishers
205 Fifth Avenue
Tarentum, Pennsylvania 15084

www.wordassociation.com

1.800.827.7903

With so much love, we would like to dedicate this book

to

Grandma, who pushed when she had to, and pulled when she needed to, but who mostly walks beside us on this journey,

and

Andy, who shows us every day the meaning of strength, resilience, and courage simply by the way he lives his life.

A note from
the authors

The stories you are about to read are the stories of our family's journey with childhood apraxia of speech. We wrote these stories over the last 15 years or so, when something moved one us or when we felt the need to take pen to paper in order to capture a moment that might otherwise be lost to the passage of time. While there were two parents in our home at the time the kids were growing up, we have chosen to focus on our family of three.

There is some repetition in our stories and they are not always in chronological order, but isn't that how memories are really?

Our stories are intended to help you, the reader, gain insight and hang on to hope throughout the process of helping your child learn to communicate in the best way possible for him or her. We are not speech-language pathologists; we are not doctors. We are in no way intending to provide medical advice to our readers.

That said, if you have concerns about your child's development in the area of speech and language, please listen to your heart. No matter how many people tell you that Albert Einstein didn't begin to speak until he was four years old. Make an appointment with a speech-language pathologist certified by the American Speech-Language-Hearing Association.

If your child has been diagnosed with childhood apraxia of speech, we urge you to visit the Childhood Apraxia of Speech Association's website at www.apraxia-kids.org. The site is free to everyone and contains the information you will need to help you help your child.

It also should be noted for the sake of disclosure that Kathy is a founding member of the Childhood Apraxia of Speech Association of North America and also serves as the Director of Education for the organization.

Kathy and Kate Hennessy

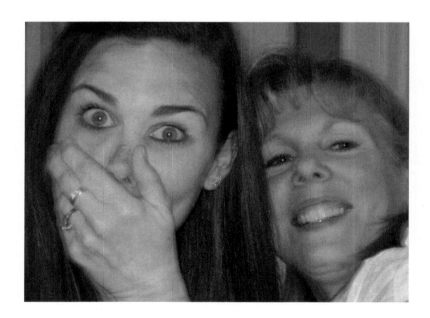

Table of Contents

Foreword

Childhood apraxia of speech (CAS) is a unique type of pediatric speech sound impairment that is characterized by a child's inability to correctly make speech sounds and smoothly blend them into words. With you as their audience, the Hennessys pull back the curtain and let you peek inside some of the events of their lives. Their lives touched by CAS. In this affecting book, they speak with a nakedness that at times feels too personal to hear, as though you're hearing things meant to stay private. You hear the difficult, the embarrassing, the ugly, the sad. You also hear the love, the care, the hope, the humor, and of their many substantial successes. The candor in their accounts left me wishing that I could stand before an audience and present with the same admirable amount of bare honesty.

Twenty years ago when Kathy was in the throes of seeking diagnoses for Kate and Andy, I was in the midst of applying to a doctoral program while working in my ninth year as a full-time clinical speech-language pathologist with my master's degree. I loved medical speech-language pathology and planned to delve into normal and disordered acquisition of speech in my doctoral studies, specializing in diagnosis and treatment of children with craniofacial abnormalities such as cleft palate; however, because of the opportunity for strong mentoring, I moved toward specializing in CAS instead. I already had clinical experience working with children with CAS and found it to be challenging, fascinating, and often frustrating work.

But 20 years ago, precisely when Kathy was hearing the word "apraxia" for the first time, there were some in my professional field who were denying the existence of CAS as a unique disorder of speech. I had not yet met the Hennessys, but I knew severe speech sound impairment and I knew that there were children who presented with a complex of motor-based symptoms that were unlike other children with speech sound impairment. Those children and their families had different needs, a correct diagnosis being just one of them. In their candidness, the Hennessys tell us of at least some of those real and often urgent needs. Family members of children with CAS will identify with the Hennessys' needs, and laugh and cry along with them. Professionals, though, have the potential to gain the most by reading this book, as it provides insight into both the depth and breadth of the needs of families affected by CAS.

Speech-language pathologists had—and continue to have—real needs, too, related to CAS. I explain to my students, largely undergraduates, that in the world of speech, language, and hearing research, CAS is low on the ladder. You see, studying speech sound impairment is not the sexiest disorder one can study. And sex appeal would not matter much if it didn't matter. But it does. It matters a lot. It matters in being able develop and fund campaigns that raise public awareness of CAS and in securing funds to conduct research. We are stymied by what we do not understand about CAS because there are so few dollars available to study it. I hope that by getting glimpses into the lives of Kathy, Kate, and Andy that readers will come to understand the importance of speech in the lives of children who have something to say, have a strong desire to say it, and work hard and for years to learn how to say it. The first child with CAS I ever worked with was five years old when I began working with her; she turned 33 years old this year. She still works hard to produce intelligible speech and she always will. Understanding speech sound impairment, including CAS, is as important as *anything* else we might direct effort and research funds to study.

If the children with CAS with whom I'm involved keep me highly motivated to continue to do this work, then their family members are the catalysts for keeping me current. As you learn in reading *Anything But Silent*, parents and other caregivers of children with CAS are very well-informed individuals. Their pursuit of answers and appropriate services for their children propel clinical and research speech-language pathologists toward learning all we can about CAS. In return, we are the recipients of some of the most devoted caregivers with whom we have the privilege of working. Like Kathy Hennessy, their high energy, and at times, their angst, spurs us to provide our very best care. We learn to respect these families and the journeys they are on.

I came to know Kathy when CASANA asked me to serve as a Professional Advisory Board Member during its formation many years ago, and ever since, my work for CASANA has been a true labor of love. I have staid respect for everyone in the organization and I'm overjoyed, but not surprised, at their tremendous success. In the chapters, *My CASANA Family* and *We Are Not Alone, We Never Were,* Kathy and Kate, respectively, talk about the importance of "the others" they brought into their lives. The Hennessys intentionally constructed within CASANA a circle of people who expanded and brought love into their family. This love helps to sustain them.

I'd like you, the reader, also to appreciate that these relationships are reciprocal. The love flows back and forth, from parent to researcher to child to staff member to family member to speech-language pathologist. Round and round it flows, sustaining all of us. It is tricky business becoming intimate with those we serve, but it's in these genuine relationships that I have found meaning for the work that I do and in the person I am. I count the Hennessys among my most treasured, my most valued, friends; indeed, we are family.

Parents and other caregivers of children with CAS, I encourage you to tell your own family's story to the professionals with whom you work, especially to your child's speech-language pathologist. For everyone involved, the CAS journey is a long one. Share *Anything But Silent* with your speech-language pathologist and talk about your own family's celebrations and struggles in an effort to build a relationship that not only will serve your child, but that best will serve you, your family members, and the professionals with whom you work. If you're searching for hope, knowledge, or a slice of humanity, you will find it within the pages of this book.

Kathy J. Jakielski, Ph.D., CCC-SLP
Florence and John Wertz Chair of the Liberal Arts and Sciences
Augustana College
Rock Island, IL

(kathy)
Living through
the diagnosis

As a parent, the diagnosis of apraxia was the most difficult part of accepting that my children were going to be different. Each time I was pregnant, I had of course imagined the perfect child that would soon be mine. The children of my imagination would never

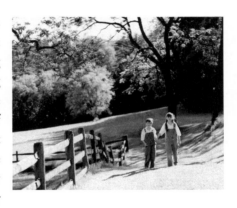

be mine. I have two children that have been diagnosed as having childhood apraxia of speech (CAS); Kate has "pure apraxia" and Andy has a total of six diagnoses of which verbal apraxia is only one. Although when I started on this odyssey I was still years away from that knowledge.

CAS is a very difficult diagnosis to understand, not just for parents, but researchers and clinicians struggle to fully grasp the intricacies of the disorder:

> Childhood apraxia of speech is a motor speech disorder.
> For reasons not yet fully understood, children with apraxia

of speech have great difficulty planning and producing the precise, highly refined and specific series of movements of the tongue, lips, jaw and palate that are necessary for intelligible speech. Apraxia of speech is sometimes called verbal apraxia, developmental apraxia of speech, or verbal dyspraxia. No matter what name is used, the most important concept is the root word "praxis." Praxis means planned movement. To some degree or another, a child with the diagnosis of apraxia of speech has difficulty programming and planning speech movements. *

Many children with CAS have motor planning difficulties in other areas as well. There is no cure. Children will not simply grow out of it. CAS is very difficult to diagnose and no one really knows why or how it occurs. Research is slowly coming along. Parents learn to speak the language of speech language pathologists as they read the medical journals searching for any information.

When Katie, my oldest, was about two years old, I was beginning to feel that something was not quite right with her speech. She was able to say "Mama" but "Dada" was too much for her. She had, on her own, developed a complex system of hand signals, gestures, and grunts to communicate with me. I patted myself on the back because she was such an intelligent child and never dreamed that the speech wouldn't come.

At the prodding of our pediatrician and without too much concern, I took her for a speech and language evaluation. She was pronounced within the parameters of "normal." I was sent home and told to come back in a year if I still felt things were not quite right.

---

* Apraxia-KIDS, 2012, Childhood Apraxia of Speech Association of North America, Family Start Guide, What is Childhood Apraxia of Speech, http://www.apraxia-kids.org.

Six months later I was back in the same office. Katie was losing some real ground socially because of her inability to communicate on the same level as her peers. The evaluation took hours. I brought the toys that Katie liked to play with best so that she could show them how well she communicated. I brought her juice and a snack. I was a totally prepared mother.

At most facilities, when you go for an evaluation, you don't leave without knowing the diagnosis. So when I sat in the office and listened as they told me my child was "developmentally delayed" my little world fell apart. It wasn't as if I had never been given bad news before...I have had a life filled with ups and downs and mountains to climb. But this was different-this was my child! As the speech pathologist continued to talk, my mind began to wander. Would Katie be able to go to college? Would she ever get married and have children of her own? What exactly were we talking about here? On one level, I was listening intently as the therapist spoke; on another level I was screaming that this was not possible for my child. I gathered together all the paperwork, all the phone numbers, and referrals that were given to me. Like a robot, I got Katie ready to go out into the cold.

A funny thing happened between the time we left the office and the time that we reached the car. I talked myself out of believing that this was so very bad. Katie would not be correctly diagnosed until she was five years old, but even then some part of my brain was denying what my heart was not ready to accept. Finally, when the written report reached our home, I could no longer deny that something was wrong and I cried and cried, and then I cried some more. Now my friends will tell you that I cry over just about anything and I cannot deny that, but I will tell you that this was different. This was the most unreachable, deepest torment I had ever experienced. The pain was so real that I could almost touch it.

Something changed that day. The child that I carried with me for nine months, the child that I told of all my hopes and dreams for her before she was even born, was gone. My unnamed dream child was gone and in her place stood reality. The reality was the bright, beautiful and engaging Katie. And Katie had a problem. I decided that day that there were two choices; I could beat my breast about the unfairness of life or I could educate myself and help my daughter move her own mountains.

I chose the second.

Then came my Andy and in my heart I knew from the day I brought him home from the hospital that something was wrong. I brought him home straight out of the intensive care unit of the hospital, where he had been for just under a week. He had aspirated meconium and developed pneumonia. I thought my fears were just left over from the scare I had during his birth and immediately afterwards. But Andy couldn't suck very well.

At this time, I had never heard of apraxia and most of my newly-acquired knowledge centered around speech delays in general and fighting insurance companies. As Andy tried to walk, I noticed that something was just a bit off. Then he stopped trying to walk altogether and it was months before he would even try again. During all this time he was completely silent. He cried, but he never babbled or made any other kind of sound. My heart was torn in half when he wouldn't kiss me. First I thought he was deaf, then I thought maybe he was autistic, then when he was 18 months old I took him for an evaluation.

I could barely get home with him. "Not again," I screamed inside myself. I just can't do this again. For the next few weeks, every time I looked at my precious little boy I cried and wondered when I was going to be able to pull myself together. The kids knew there was something wrong with Mommy. What they didn't know was that Mommy cried for them. Mommy was crying because she had seen what Katie had to go through, lost playtime due to hours of therapy; frustration when no one, not even Mom, could understand what she was trying to say; and tears when she couldn't make Barbie talk. Mommy cried because she knew that even though there was no definitive diagnosis, Andy would now travel that same road.

Andy was not diagnosed with apraxia until almost a year later and then Katie, who was five years old and in kindergarten, was diagnosed with apraxia. The final piece of the puzzle would fall into place and some things finally became clear. It wasn't that Andy wouldn't give Mommy a kiss, but that Andy couldn't give Mommy a kiss.

I think having gone through this twice now I have learned something. I think that we have to allow ourselves to grieve for what we have lost, even if it was only a dream. We as parents need to understand that it is okay to cry and be upset and rail against the unfairness of life. Acceptance is a process and we must allow ourselves to go through that process. I think we must ask why and all the other questions that cannot possibly be answered. Then and only then can we pick up the pieces and do what is best for our children.

I also believe that in having lost what wasn't real to begin with I was given a chance to accept my children as they truly are. Parents of teenagers go through this, too. Suddenly the child who just a short time ago would do anything to please you has a mind of her own and a personality to go with it. Just as the parent of a budding teenager must accept that the beautiful child sulking in her bedroom with her pierced eyebrow was never meant to be the child you imagined, I, as the parent of children with disabilities had to learn to accept my kids for who and what they really were. My children are more than a diagnosis that has been assigned to them. Our children are shining examples of spirits that cannot be broken. They are the modern-day heroes that others are so desperately seeking. They will be the truly compassionate adults of the future, because they will know what it is to move a mountain. And someday they may want to pierce something, too.

Seven years have gone by since Katie was first diagnosed, five years for Andy, and as I finish writing this, I can hear the sounds of Katie and Andy playing school downstairs. They are there with a few of their friends. I know that there is still work to be done for both of them, but as I strain to listen I can hear their voices, but I can't tell my children from any of the other children and I believe I am going to cry again.

(k a t e)
My future begins
in the past

Becasue I wasn't the parent sitting in the room being told there was something wrong with my child, being diagnosed with apraxia means something entirely different to me than it does to my mother.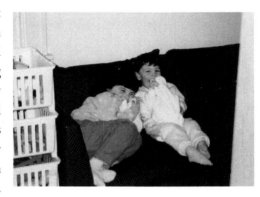
I never had to go through the grieving process of letting go of the dreams of a certain type of parenthood.

What I do think about though is the future. To place the end at the beginning, so to speak, when I think back to being diagnosed with apraxia, I think of my future. When I grow up and decide whether or not to have kids, will those kids have apraxia? Will the roles be reversed and will I have to go through everything my mom did? Would it be wrong to even have children, knowing that their future could possibly be filled with constant speech therapy, the outcome really unknown?

There are so many mysteries when looking into the future and thinking about apraxia, but I can't help thinking about it. I also can't help thinking about the man I decide to settle down with. Couples discuss the possibility of children while they are dating, but how do you explain a future that could be filled with IEP's, speech therapy, and constant challenges to some unsuspecting guy.

There are probably not too many twenty-year-olds who would be able to wrap their head around what that really means. Would a young adult really even understand what a crapshoot it is to have a child? Is anyone prepared to have a child with a disability? Apraxia, though rare, doesn't seem to be as uncommon as first thought. "Pure apraxia," which is the type of apraxia I have, is rare. "Pure apraxia" affects only a person's speech. He or she would have no other issues. In the world of apraxia it is pretty uncommon for someone with apraxia not to be diagnosed with other issues, too. In addition to "speech apraxia," Andy is also diagnosed with "global apraxia" that affects the control he has over muscles all over his body. He also has other diagnoses that influence his life. I have to ask myself, how can two kids from the same family, with a similar diagnosis, be so different? What kinds of issues would my kids have, if any?

What about the money it takes to have a child with issues? I know that having a child is a huge financial commitment to begin with, but add in the cost of speech therapy 3 or 4 times a week for 7-12 years and the numbers become overwhelming. I recognize the constant battles with insurance companies and the toll that it takes on a parent.

I suppose in some ways I have the advantage in that I really do "get" all this; I understand. I understand what it takes to work hard to achieve something that comes so easily to everyone else. But how do you have this conversation with your partner? How do you make him understand any of it? I pray Mr. Wonderful of the future just doesn't say, "It will all be fine," because I know that sometimes it just isn't. Will Mr. Right even want to be with me after hearing all that? Whoever Prince Charming turns to be, he better be up for the challenge. I have a lot I want to do in my life before any of this matters, but as someone who is diagnosed with apraxia, I can't help but think about it sometimes.

While we've come so far in the past two decades, it seems like there is still much to discover about apraxia in children. Whenever asked, I will always participate in research about apraxia. I feel like it's my responsibility to the children who come after me and to the children who may be mine in the future.

Having a child with apraxia is a struggle of epic proportions, but there are still things in the world that are worse. There are still many questions that do not have answers, but for most children with apraxia it will get better, like it did for me. My battles with apraxia are finished now and I am living all the secret dreams I used to think would be impossible for a kid like me. So, to my little rug rats of the future that may have apraxia I say, "Keep those jelly hands off the furniture and game on!"

(kathy)

First words:
When you know that
he will talk

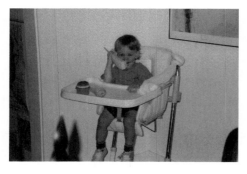

"Kathy, you need to prepare yourself for the very real possibility that he may never speak at all. Your miracle may very well be that he can walk." The tide roared in my head. I couldn't think. I couldn't breathe. Nothing would ever be the same again for three-year-old Andy. Was this how it felt to die...just a little?

I had done this before, with Katie. I knew what I had to do. I had to get everything back in the bag. Find my keys. Don't cry in front of the therapist. Put Andy in the car seat. Get home without wrecking the car. It would be okay. Andy could use sign language to communicate. I would hire someone to teach the whole family. He would communicate. Put the car in reverse. Don't hit the car behind. Now forward. Look right, left, now turn. What if he never talked? Don't think about that, just drive. How can I do this again?

Stop at the light. Look in the rearview mirror. Who is that woman? Why does she look so scared? Oh, it's me. Just drive. Think later.

I wish I could not remember how those first few days after Andy's diagnosis of childhood apraxia of speech felt. But I remember every minute, every second. I refuse to let it go. I refuse to forget. I want to remember so that I will know how far we have come. Andy made no speech sounds. He had never made any sounds like babbling. He was in therapy for a year and still there were no real sounds. I cannot remember what tests they gave Andy when he first started therapy at eighteen months, but when they tested him a year later with the same tests, his scores were worse than when we started therapy-that's what I remember. Apraxia was what she said. I had never heard that word before. I didn't know what it meant.

When I took him to preschool the next day, I sat in a corner with Karen Frank, his teacher, and Louise Foster, the director of the school. Apraxia. Maybe he'll never talk. They cried, too. We talked for a long time. Louise and Karen believed he would talk. They never doubted. They made a safe place for Andy while I figured out this apraxia. I started to read. I read anything I could get my hands on. Education, that was going to be the answer to apraxia.

I made Plan "A". I would give therapy six months. If Andy didn't start at least making some kind of speech sounds in six months, then I would go to Plan "B." Plan "B" was to hire an American Sign Language teacher to teach Andy and our extended family sign language. One way or the other, Andy would communicate.

In the meantime, I would teach Andy and myself enough sign language so that I could at least communicate with him a little. I bought *The Joy of Signing*. I couldn't decide where to start. How about colors? Five words a day; that was how we started. Blue, yellow, red, white, and black, I had no idea that Andy knew his colors. I felt horrible. How could he know his colors and I not know that? I was the worst mother on earth. By the time Andy was three-and-a-half years old, he knew over 250 words. As fast as I could learn it and pass it on, that's how fast he could learn it. I found out something else about Andy, he was funny. And sometimes it was a good thing he was signing or it would have been embarrassing.

What about Plan "A?" All the while Andy was learning to sign, he was also trying to learn to speak. He went into speech therapy five times a week. I learned how to work with him at home. I learned how to fight with my insurance company. I learned not to care what other people thought as they watched us sign and talk at the same time. I learned that my little boy was really smart. And I waited for a sound. At this point, it wasn't as if Andy didn't make any sounds at all. From the time he woke up in the morning until the time he went to bed at night, he made the sound of the siren of a fire engine. No matter where we were or who we were with, he screeched like a siren. It drove me to the brink of madness as I waited for a speech sound. I called my friend Patty and made arrangements for her to teach us American Sign Language at the end of the six months. And I waited.

Finally, it started to happen. It turns out there was no red letter day, no moment where I knew we had turned a corner. No flash of intuition when I knew we had our real miracle. The knowledge came with hard work, determination, patience, and absolute faith in my child. The knowledge came not with "mama" or "dada," but with a "mmmm" and a smile. I called Patty and told her I didn't think we would need those lessons after all. Andy was three-and-a-half and he said "mmm." It was enough for me.

There was more therapy. There was always more therapy, no breaks, no vacations, just therapy. There was more to say than just "mmm." When Katie started therapy, she went five times a week, two of those sessions lasted two-and-a-half hours each. From the very beginning, she got the connection between going to "talking practice" and talking to her friends. She also really enjoyed the one-on-one sessions with an adult. Andy, on the other hand, was content to be at home playing with his LEGO or Brio blocks. He didn't enjoy the whole concept of going out, he still doesn't. He never liked therapy. He never wanted to go. He never "got it." He just wanted to stay home and play. Looking back, I think Andy was the more typical child and Katie the anomaly, but at the time it was a struggle. Katie liked to practice at home. She liked the idea of having me all to herself. Andy liked the idea of playing with his LEGO. So I had to get creative. I was never able to just go at the therapy head on; I had to hide it in the LEGO and the Brio. As long as it didn't look like therapy, Andy was happy to comply. Apraxia became a way of life for us. We practiced at home in the tub, while getting dinner, and while sorting laundry. We practiced in the car and in the grocery store. We practiced whenever there was an opportunity to talk. Whatever sound we were working on was never far from my thoughts. Soon Andy had a repertoire of sounds. He had no words, but he had speech sounds. We were moving along.

When Andy started to make those first few sounds it was like Mardi Gras in our house. When Katie was nine-years-old she was dismissed from therapy after seven long years. We went to Disneyland. Okay, we were going to go anyway, but we celebrated all through Disneyland. High fives, hugs, and McFlurry's were common after a good hour of therapy.

When did I really know that it was all going to work out for Andy? There was never a watershed moment in time when the future was suddenly crystal clear and sailing became smooth, but by the end of kindergarten it was clear to all of us that Andy was going to be able to speak in some manner. The clarity of his speech would be in question for many years to come, but he was trying, making progress, and accomplishing his goals.

(kate)

Journeys

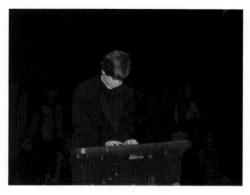

Learning sign language gave Andy and me a way to communicate on a very basic level. Finally, while we were learning to talk, we had a way to convey our wants and needs to our mom. It can be very frustrating to get apple juice when what you really wanted was orange juice. So just being able to communicate the most basic things was an unimaginable relief for everyone. Sign language was how we communicated in our house for a very long time.

But my mom was living in two different worlds and she had to find a way to make them meet in the middle. My mom came from the theater world, a world based on communication, and now she was living in a world where communication was the most difficult, if not impossible thing. Her world was full of contradictions.

Through our elementary school PTA my mom met another woman who would give her the way to let it all make sense. Aileen Owens had an idea and she began a journey all her own. The school-based program she created, Journeys, was a collaboration involving local businesses, universities, working professionals, parents, and teachers that provided really unique, hands-on learning opportunities for children that didn't exist in public school education. So, in the fall of 1996 when I was in first grade, my mom, and another woman who had also worked in theater and had children at our elementary school, began to teach the thing that they were passionate about: theater. Andy and I grew up in what is often referred to as a "walking community." There are seven elementary schools in our district, one within walking distance of each home. We had a full-hour lunch period as most of the kids did walk home for lunch. On theater days, 25 of us packed a lunch, met in the gym, and began "Building a Character in Time," as the theater program was called.

Everyone loved the theater class and it was always full, but my mom was already thinking ahead and thinking about something different. She was still cogitating about the two worlds she was living in and trying to figure out a way to bring them together. The first year of the theater program Andy was still in preschool and the second year of the program he was not at our home school. He was in the speech and language classroom in another building, but he was going to Lincoln Elementary and Mom was determined to find a way for him to be in her class. When she finally figured it out, she called her program "Connections."

In the Connections program we studied the history of the Deaf culture and then we created characters and wrote scripts based on our research. We worked with Carnegie Mellon University, The Western Pennsylvania School for the Deaf, and the National Theater of the Deaf; and through our mentors we learned the scripts we wrote in sign language.

"Building a Character in Time" and "Connections" provided so many opportunities, not just for me, but for all the kids involved. Through the years that my mom taught theater, I played a Greek goddess, a young girl working in the factories during the Industrial Revolution, a basketball player who just happened to be deaf, and Sarah, a young girl living during the Civil War whose friendship with one of her family's slaves is tested. We studied history, and learned sign language. Because we wrote our own scripts it was entirely up to us to do the research that went into creating our own characters.

The role that still stands out for me is Helen Keller. As a fourth grader, Helen's story inspired me as we shared the inability to communicate with the people that we loved. As it turned out I would much rather speak to a room of hundreds of adults about apraxia rather than act on a stage in front of my peers.

Mom wrote a connecting narrative that made all the kids scripts into one big story. We always ended our show with a song we choreographed and also learned in sign language. So many people told my mom that it would be impossible for kids to do all the things she was asking from them. Everything the nay-sayers said couldn't be done with kids, we did.

The thing about Connections was that it mixed kids from all grade levels and abilities. No kid who wanted to be a part of Connections was ever turned away. My mom had only one rule that we all had to live by: no matter what happened on the playground or in the classroom, in that gym we were all friends and we all supported and rooted for each other. If you couldn't live with just this one rule you had to deal with my mother. For the most part, it was a different world in that gym twice a week.

Connections threw together kids with all kinds of disabilities and kids with no disabilities. We got to know everyone and because we were focused on our scripts and learning them in sign language, and with learning our song and choreography we forgot to notice the things that made us different from each other.

Connections made sign language "cool" in our school. Andy and I suddenly knew something that all the other kids wanted to know. Finally, we were the cool kids and we had something to share with our friends. And that really goes double for little girls. Little girls love the idea of having a secret language that no one else knows and I was the one who could show them how to talk with their hands. For so very long I had struggled to feel like I was part of the group and at last I had something that everybody else wanted.

And that was the thing about Connections, it gave us confidence. We all had our private struggles, but at the end of our time together we would each get up on the stage and perform in front of a few hundred people, including our classmates and families. Even Andy, whose speech issues were so much more severe than mine took his place onstage and performed the script that he wrote and signed along with it. He was fearless.

And when Connections was all wrapped up for the year, we went back to our places on the playground with a new-found appreciation for the kid on the other side of the field. We might not be best friends, but we understood each other's struggle and the strength that each of us really had inside. And finally, my mom found a way to put her worlds together into one wonderful show. Her unwavering belief that we were all capable of doing more than anyone thought possible led us on a journey to understanding, compassion, and tolerance.

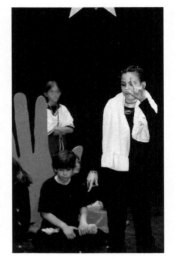

There is more going on here than I thought!

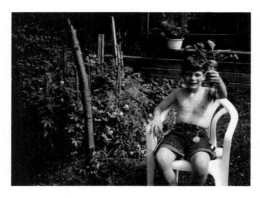

By the time Andy entered first grade, he had already received the primary diagnosis of childhood apraxia of speech, along with diagnoses of global apraxia, sensory integration disorder (SID), hypotonia, and attention deficit hyperactivity disorder (ADHD). I felt though that there was still something missing from the picture that I couldn't quite put my finger on and it puzzled me. It was in fourth grade that Andy was diagnosed with obsessive compulsive disorder (OCD) that presented itself as hoarding-and another piece of the Andy puzzle fell into place. Finally, in high school, Andy would receive the final diagnosis of Social Anxiety Disorder. "Well duh," I thought, "If I had all that other stuff going on, I would be anxious, too!"

After Andy was born he was discharged right from the NICU to home. I begged the hospital not to send him home so quickly because I had no idea what to do with a kid who had been that ill.

But he came home and so began the odyssey of trying to figure out what was up with Andy.

A couple things about Andy became evident right off the bat and thankfully my mother was there to help. Andy just wouldn't sleep in his crib. I tried everything: I swaddled him, I played the musical mobile, I made the room quiet, I left the lights on to mimic the NICU, I turned the lights off. Nothing worked and Andy cried every time I put him in the crib. The poor guy was just exhausted. It was my mom who came up with the winning idea of swaddling him and laying him in the molded plastic baby seat and putting the seat in the crib. Andy finally slept and so did I. Looking back, it's clear to me now that it was Andy's sensory issues that were at the heart of the problem. Once we wrapped him tightly and put him in that seat where he could feel the sides around him limiting his space, he was happy. Was this an indication of the sensory issues that would loom over Andy's life in the years to come?

After I finally got Andy to sleep I couldn't get him to wake up! It would take me well over an hour to feed him a bottle. Again, I tried everything to get him to suck his bottle, up to and including taking a pin to make the hole in the nipple a little bigger. After finally getting most of the bottle in him, Andy would sleep until it was time for the next bottle. It worried me, a lot. Finally, I decided to call the pediatrician. Wow, that was a mistake! The doctor really made me feel like an idiot with comments like, "Well, most mothers would kill for a baby that slept like that!" and "What exactly do you want me to do?" Yikes! So Andy and I muddled through and I started him on oatmeal mixed with formula at six weeks. The kid was hungry and he couldn't suck. Looking back, Andy's inability to suck was a loud and clear red flag that there was some kind of motor planning problem. Ah, if I knew then what I know now.

All those red flags and Andy was in high school before I had a complete picture of what the issues were that complicated his life. But I knew, and I knew from day one, that there was a lot going on with Andy. Life with Andy was always interesting as he developed his own strategies to cope with the undiagnosed disorders. He loved rocks and every rock he saw during any given day became his most very favorite rock of all time, and he had to have the rock with him in his bedroom. It got a little hard to dust and I needed to get the darn rocks out of the house. Finally when Andy was around six or seven years old, I put a couple of baskets by the front door and Andy had to empty his pockets before he came in the house. When the baskets got full we would empty them in the garden. It was a good deal for Andy and it sure made cleaning his room easier. Although there were still the McDonald's paper placemats that always had to be brought home and always ended up in Andy's bedroom. I came up with elaborate reasons as to why Andy seemed to need all this stuff in his room; something about needing to take something from one environment into the next in order to feel okay. But whatever, the bedroom was still a mess. What I did learn was that once the stuff hit his room, Andy didn't really care what happened to it. So every once in a while when Andy wasn't around, I would sneak in his room with a garbage bag and clean it out. That went on until Andy left for college; sometimes he noticed and sometimes he didn't.

Andy also couldn't walk down the hallway in the house without knocking the pictures off the wall. I had to replace the glass in those pictures every couple of months. It was the worst when Andy came home from school after he had been sitting all day. On some days the kids would head straight to the swing set before coming into the house from school. I noticed on those days that Andy seemed more in control of his body. So I began to routinely send him out to swing on the swing set before he came into the house. The swinging seemed to calm his body and let him walk through the house without losing his balance and falling too much. When we stood in any line, he had to have family members in front of and behind him so that he would not stomp on too many people's feet.

Andy was cute and cuddly and loved to play with his sister and me and we had great fun, but always lurking beneath the surface were the questions. I knew there was much more going on with him, I just couldn't put all the pieces together and it frustrated the heck out of me. At the same time, I'm not really sure it would have made all that much difference to have the full picture from the beginning. What I mean is how much can a kid really work on all at once anyway? The most important thing for Andy when he was preschool age and even into early elementary was to learn to speak, plain and simple. The physical therapy, the occupational therapy, the equestrian therapy were all well and good, but speech therapy was the primary focus. As Andy became a verbal communicator, the focus changed to working on the pragmatic skills he missed perfecting while he focused on learning to speak. A child who can't talk misses learning the give-and-take of play and sometimes that results in even more therapy to catch him up to his peers. His balance and sensory issues also were tackled later in elementary school. We really dealt with Andy's social anxiety in high school and honestly, getting out of high school and going to college was the best thing that ever happened to Andy.

So does that mean that all kids with childhood apraxia of speech are going to have a whole host of other issues? Not necessarily. Kate has CAS and absolutely no other issues, and she wrapped up her therapy by the end of third grade. She had no real academic support after she was dismissed from speech therapy. That said, it does seem more often than not children that who have been diagnosed with CAS seem to be vulnerable to other neurologic issues. If you see a red flag and something about your child's development is bothering you, go have that evaluation done. If the doctor tries to make you feel silly or like you're overreacting, go somewhere else! You are the person who knows your child best and you are the only person who will fight for your child. You are the person your child depends on and someday, hopefully with his own voice, he will thank you!

Around the corner,
around the country

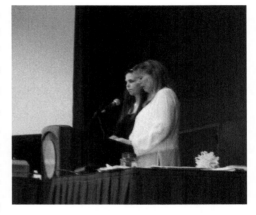

I am different than Andy. I am so different than Andy it's sometimes hard to remember that we come from the same mother. While Andy's apraxia is complicated by many other issues, I have what is referred to as "pure" apraxia. I have no other diagnosed neurological issues. While there was some question as to whether Andy would ever have the ability to speak, there was never any doubt I would talk. The quality of my speech was what was in question in the beginning. Would Kate ever have intelligible speech? Would anyone ever be able to understand Kate when she spoke? These questions haunted my mother from early on.

Once I did learn to speak clearly, I never stopped. Teachers never really understood that the notes they sent home telling my mother that I talked all the time, in class and out of class, were cause for celebration and I was never once reprimanded for doing the thing we had all worked so hard to accomplish.

So, in 2004 when my mother and I were invited to help out and also speak at a CASANA workshop, it seemed like it would be a task that was right up my alley. But I was in seventh grade and at that point being just like all my classmates was really important to me. It had been a long time since I had been in speech therapy and I had worked very hard to separate apraxia from my life as a teenager. It didn't take much to convince me that I wanted to go, though. I think my mom had me at, "Do you want to travel to..." Before I knew it, we were on our way to Fairfax, Virginia for our first apraxia workshop.

Putting my mom and me in a car together is always an adventure and trying to navigate our way through the Washington Beltway was as entertaining as it gets. But in the end, we made it to Fairfax. We met up with the folks who organized the workshop and jumped into the chaos of attempting to put everything together. As the day went on it became clear that this workshop was not going to go exactly as planned. With over 100 attendees, a room set for 80 just wasn't going to work. From then on, everything that could go wrong, did.

By the end of that first day I had met many people that I would become close to in the years that followed, including Dr. Edythe Strand from the Mayo Clinic in Rochester, Minnesota. Dr. Strand is considered one of our nation's leading experts in the field of childhood apraxia of speech. Beyond that, she has turned out to be one of the finest people I have ever known. The extent of Edy's knowledge and understanding about childhood apraxia of speech is obvious when you listen to her lecture. Her passion for children with apraxia is also evident. Yet, Edy remains down-to-earth and reachable, and it's clear how much she loves us.

It was a two-day workshop and mom and I were scheduled to speak on the first day. We woke up extremely early to help make sure that everything was ready by the time the first attendee arrived. It's a good thing because our lecture hall was just a big empty room, no tables, no chairs, no screen or audio visual equipment and no breakfast. With only an hour to go until the lecture was to begin, we were in full crisis mode. Everyone was lugging chairs into a room that was never going to be large enough. And early arrivals were pressed into service helping set up the breakfast. Once Dr. Strand began the lecture I thought the worst was over. I was so wrong! About an hour into the workshop a loud bang stopped everything. The microphones were buzzing so loud that no one could hear her. The thing with Edy is, micro-phoned or not, she is fabulous and the audience was just happy to be there with her.

Marcia Robinson was the person who was organizing the workshop on behalf of CASANA, and even though that was the first time I had met her, I knew that we were going to be friends. She was always able to make me laugh, especially in the middle of a crisis, and that is exactly what she did in Fairfax. Marcia made a memorable first impression!

About an hour before lunch was supposed to start on that first day, we realized that the food was once again missing. We tried to find Marcia to let her know the latest crisis. The kitchen was in a building right next to the lecture hall and Marcia, unbeknownst to us, had marched across the alley to find the boxed lunches. We heard Marcia before we actually saw her. Mom and I stepped into the alley and all we could see was Marcia's backend sticking out of the kitchen door while she was confronting the people in the kitchen as to the whereabouts of lunch for our group. I don't think I ever laughed so hard. I felt sorry for the guys that had to face the front of her that day. I knew in that moment that we would share many adventures with Marcia and I looked forward to every crazy workshop to come.

After lunch, suddenly it was my turn and my stomach dropped. There were a lot of people in that room! Mom and I walked to the front of the room and all the people were looking at me, smiling. The smiling made everything worse, it was like an audience of happy dolls getting ready to attack. First we showed a video that we had put together showing the different stages of my apraxia. Because of my speech today, people were pretty shocked to know that the little girl in the video who struggled to speak was me. Every time little Katie on the screen started to sing I tried to hide in my seat. Somehow, my seven-year-old self thought I was the next Britney Spears.

Finally, the video was over and I crawled out from under my chair. As Mom stood and started to make her way to the podium, I wondered if I might be able to escape out the back. One look from Mom and I quickly realized there was nowhere to go but with her in front of all of those smiling faces. My mom started to talk and that meant that I would have to say something soon as well. I could not look at people when I spoke. It was so awkward and made me forget what it was I was supposed to say. I looked at the back wall while I was "speechifying," as my Mom liked to call it.

Toward the end of my speech, I think I actually started to enjoy it and I know I snuck a look or two at the audience. But it seemed as soon as it started it was over, even though it lasted more than a half an hour. I looked at my mom after we had gone to the back of the room and started smiling, a lot! I had done it! With my mom right by my side, I had shared my story in front of over one hundred people! That was more people than my entire middle school. I was so excited that for weeks afterward I couldn't stop talking about it with my mom. "When can we do it again?" "Can we go someplace even cooler?" "Mom, that was so awesome wasn't it?" "I totally want to do this again!" How my mom got through that drive home, I will never know!

After the workshop in Fairfax my mom and I continued to speak at CASANA workshops and conferences. By January of 2006, I was sixteen-years-old and my mom was organizing and running the workshops for CASANA and we were headed to Phoenix, Arizona. By that time, Mom and I had come to the realization that perhaps it was time for me to start doing that part of the workshop on my own, so I presented my story solo for the first time. Even when I didn't speak at a workshop or conference, I would attend to volunteer and help out, and I still do whenever possible.

I have met some truly remarkable people in the years that I have been volunteering for CASANA. I like spending time with them and I am so thankful for the work they do to help children with apraxia like Andy and me. CASANA has made such huge strides in making people aware of childhood apraxia of speech and all of these people have played a crucial role in advancing that understanding.

As grateful as I am for all of these researchers and speech therapists, it's truly the parents that make attending the workshops and conferences special for me. I can only imagine what it felt like for my mom when she was told both of her children may never speak. We were diagnosed at a time when, if you put 'apraxia' in the search engine on the internet, nothing would come up. When Andy and I were diagnosed, we did not even have a home computer. My mom felt so isolated and alone, wondering if her children were the only ones dealing with this rare disorder. Every parent that I meet has his or her own story, but the stories all have common threads. I want to hear about the journey that each family is making and I hope that meeting me helps them see there is a voice waiting for their child on the other side of all the therapy.

But it's not just the parents, either. A few years ago I went to a fundraiser for CASANA. I met a young girl around eleven or twelve years old; she had apraxia and was super shy. It took a long time for my mom and me to draw her out and get her to start talking to us. Pretty soon though, she was comfortable and began to open up to us. She said that she had never met another person with apraxia and she was so excited to be able to meet me and talk to me. It dawned on me then that I was so used to growing up with Andy that I didn't realize that most children with apraxia aren't lucky enough to have a brother or sister with the same disorder. Other kids spend their childhood fighting apraxia and don't know one single other person with the same disorder. It makes a difference. That's why I share my story.

The word 'hope' comes up a lot at the conferences and workshops. Hope for the future. Hope for happiness. Hope for children who struggle. It makes me sad that parents sometimes feel hopeless in the long battle they face with their children. We have come so far since Andy and I were diagnosed; no parents should have to feel the way that my mom did ever again. There are conferences and workshops now, webinars, support groups and the Apraxia-Kids website that has hundreds of pages of information just waiting to be read.

Even with all that in place, there are few places a parent can go to hear the story of one family's journey, and so I share my story with the hope that I can make even one family's worry a little less. My mom had absolutely no idea what the future held for Andy and me. She had no way of even guessing what the future might look like for us. Apraxia is different in every child, and the outcome for every child will be different, but I still think it's important for parents to see what resolved apraxia can look like. All I ever wanted when I was in the middle of all this was to be like every other kid. Finally, that's where I am.

Two special children, many choices

Second place winner of the St. Mary's College Meekison 1999 Essay Contest

Choices...When I was a teenager I thought my big choice in life was, "Should I cut my hair or let it grow?" The first real choice in my life was where would I go to college? I don't remember my family

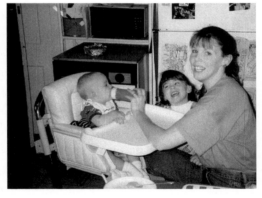

trying to sway me in any direction, but I'm still not sure how much "choice" was really involved, either. It was almost 24 years ago that I first drove up the "Avenue" at the entrance to St. Mary's. It was like coming home to a place I had never been. It was fate! I knew this was going to be "my school." This was my "choice."

As I got older, I came to believe that fate or destiny made our choices for us. We were just careening down life's path, being tossed hither and yon at the whim of some magical force. But then again, I was in my twenties.

When I was thirty-one I had my first child and it wasn't until I was pregnant with my second child that I began to face that fact that something was not quite right with my baby! I have always been the type of person to trust my instincts and did the same this time. From that point in time it took almost five years to correctly diagnose my daughter's issues and even then it was my second child, my son, who was diagnosed first. He was easier to diagnose because his issues were much more severe.

Is it fate, or destiny, or some choice we made earlier in life that sends us one of God's special children? How about two? Both of my children were eventually diagnosed with apraxia. Because very little research has been done on the issue there is not much known about apraxia. What we do know is that it is a motor planning or programming problem. Simply put, the correct message in the child's brain doesn't quite make it to the appropriate muscles to carry out the job. Apraxia often shows up in a child's speech, like in my daughter, or it can show up globally, in all the motor systems, like in my son. Researchers do not know why it occurs or what the outcome will be. There are a variety of characteristics and not every child has every characteristic, and recovery is different for every child! Researchers haven't quite figured out what to do about it, either. So, as parents, we are left to make the choices for our children with incomplete information.

As the shock of my daughter's initial and, as it turned out incorrect, diagnosis wore off, I had no idea what the future would hold for her. But the crying had to stop and I rolled up my sleeves and went to work. Katie was soon in therapy every day of the week. I was becoming an expert in fighting with insurance companies and winning, and she was learning how to speak. Looking back the most important choice I made during that period was to fight this thing, whatever "it" was.

I still didn't know how it would all turn out for Katie, when I began to realize that my son, Andy, had some issues of his own! He never did get the hang of sucking and made absolutely no sounds at all! And the thing that broke my heart the most was that he wouldn't give me kisses. At eighteen months old Andy started therapy without a diagnosis. Even though I knew he wasn't deaf, I started to teach him sign language. It was unbearably sad for me to realize all the things that were locked in Andy's head that he couldn't share with us. About a year later, Andy was diagnosed with apraxia.

Katie's therapists, at that point, diagnosed her as having severe verbal apraxia. Sadness permeated everything that I tried to do. I could not function. Choices? I felt like any choices I had were ripped from my hands and shredded to nothing. It was only later that I realized that parents of children diagnosed with disabilities must allow themselves time to grieve. There is a loss and it has to be acknowledged. But there also comes a point where choices must be made. My choice was education.

Over the years, I have often wondered what I would do if God suddenly appeared in my kitchen and offered to change my children. I have thought about this a lot and I think I would have to politely refuse His very generous offer. I believe that my children are kinder, more thoughtful, and better people for all the trials they have had to endure. Katie and Andy always take the new child in class under their wing. They tend to look out for the kids that are different from them. I don't think I taught them that; the lives they have led have been their best teachers.

What I needed at this point in my life, more than anything, was another parent and that was the one thing I couldn't find. Was it fate that sent me to just one more conference? Well, fate, destiny, or choice, it was a turning point. I found myself in a room full of parents with children just like mine. I missed the entire first hour of the conference looking around marveling at all the other parents, just like me. After the conference I introduced myself to the organizers.

Together, we have opened the doors for many other parents and because of the organization that has been formed, The Apraxia Parent Network, parents of a child newly-diagnosed with apraxia never have to feel as alone as I did in those early days. My choice in all of this has been to share my experiences and the information I have acquired along the way with other parents. Both of my children are well on the road to recovery. Katie wants nothing more than to be in a movie with Mary Kate and Ashley Olsen and Andy is an incredibly intelligent and articulate little boy who dreams of building his own amusement park one day.

Choices...when I was young I used to pray that God would solve my problems for me. As I have grown older, I have begun to pray that God helps me make good choices and gives me the 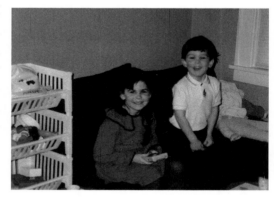 strength to see them through. It is the choices that we make that lead us to the turning points in our lives. Fate, destiny, choices, someday when I have the time I'm going to think about that and try to figure out which has had the bigger voice in my life.

(kate)

Overcoming the odds

First place winner of the August Wilson Essay Contest April, 2007. This essay also appears on the Apraxia-Kids website, www. apraxia-kids.org

One Microphone: $250. A Wooden Podium: $300. Speaking for the first time in front of a room filled with more than one hundred people listening to every word you say: Priceless. I had 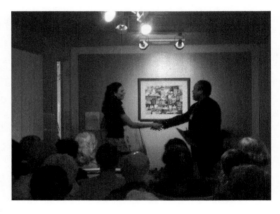 been asked to speak at a workshop held in Fairfax, Virginia when I was in seventh grade, about four years ago. The workshop was on childhood apraxia of speech, a very rare neurological speech disorder that affects between one to five children in every one thousand, www.apraxia-kids.org. I had been asked to speak in

Fairfax because not only am I diagnosed with CAS, but after seven years of intensive speech therapy, my apraxia is resolved.

In a person who is not diagnosed with apraxia of speech, the messages from his or her brain travels to the muscles in their mouth signaling how to move them in order to form words. However, with a child diagnosed with CAS, those same messages never reach the muscles, and so the child has to be taught the correct positions, for each and every sound, how to move his mouth in order to form words. What comes naturally to children learning how to speak is something that is very difficult to a child with apraxia.

When I was two and a half years old, I was diagnosed as "developmentally delayed." As the years have gone by, I've realized that this diagnosis is often given to people when the doctors know something is not quite right, but cannot seem to find exactly what is wrong with that person. After a few years, I was finally correctly diagnosed with childhood apraxia of speech after my younger brother was first diagnosed with it. I was five years old. From the time I was two, I went to speech therapy five days a week while other kids played outside. Practicing my speech however was not something confined to the therapist's office. We practiced everywhere. From the car, to the grocery store, anywhere you could think of, we practiced speech there.

It might seem as if my childhood revolved around speech therapy, and it did, to an extent. But I was still a regular kid who had tons of fun. My mom made it her mission to make sure that my brother and I were always having fun, no matter how many times we had to practice our vowel sounds. Speech therapy was just another thing in our lives and because of this, it never really stuck out to me. The way I like to think of it is that people tend to remember the big things in their lives, the things that really stick out, like graduations, birthdays, vacations. Speech therapy never seemed like it was a

hassle or something that made us different. In August Wilson's
Fences he says, "Death ain't nothing but a fastball on the outside
corner." Apraxia was not something that made me feel different
from all the other kids. It was just another mountain to climb, or
a fastball in the corner. I do not even really remember that much
concerning therapy, well, besides the tons of ice cream we would
always get from the McDonald's across the street after therapy.

Apraxia is something that will never go away. Though I am
resolved today, it still affects so many different aspects of my life.
I stumble on words here and there, but after I hear how the word
is correctly pronounced, it seems to stay with me. One of the
words I remember having immense difficulty with as a child was
cemetery. That word took me days to learn how to pronounce.
I remember sitting on my bed at night with my mother working
through the word backwards, something that seems to work best
for children with apraxia, trying to learn how to say it correctly.
Once I had the word down, it felt like the biggest accomplishment
because of how long it had taken me to learn it. Another word was
"archipelago." Funny thing is though, my mother thought it was
pronounced a different way that it truly was, and so to this day I
always say it the way I learned it because that is how my muscles
in my mouth were taught from the start.

Since that fateful first speech in Fairfax, I've been given the
opportunity to speak at ten different events, ranging from
workshops, parent meetings, and even national conferences, in
nine different cities across the country. The first few times I spoke,
my mother and I did a presentation together. I would always end
up having to kick her under the podium in the hopes of reminding
her that crying while speaking in front of people probably was not
the best decision, no matter if she could help it or not!

I look at my success at having overcome apraxia as a responsibility to inspire people, to give hope when it seems as if it is lost. When both my brother and I were diagnosed with CAS, my mother felt alone, as if she was the only parent going through all of the struggles because it seemed as if no one had ever heard of apraxia. I don't want any other parent to ever feel that way, and so I have made it my mission to make sure that parents know that there is a future in store for their kids, a future that does not include speech therapy every day of the week. I look at myself as an advocate for children with disabilities, and stick up for them when others do not truly understand what it feels like to have to work so hard for something that comes so easy for many. August Wilson states in *Joe Turner's Come and Gone,* "Everybody has to find his own song. Now, I can look at you, Mr. Loomis, and see you a man who done forgot his song. Forgot how to sing it. A fellow forget that and he forget who he is. Forget how he's supposed to mark down life...See, Mr. Loomis, when a man forgets his song, he goes off in search of it...till he find out he's got it with him all the time." I have found my song in life, and that is to inspire people and give hope when all else seems impossible. I've embraced all that there is about apraxia, because it is a part of who I am, no matter what I do. I would never wish apraxia was not part of my life. It has made me a more sensitive, aware, and caring person. I do not look at people and make judgments, because no one can truly get to know a person from the outside; it is their inside, their soul that truly matters.

I've met some truly amazing people and have even become friends with some of the top researchers in apraxia in the entire country. I have so much respect for these professionals, because of all their dedication in helping kids like me gain a voice, and families, who never give up on their children. Like these incredible researchers and families, August Wilson was able to achieve greatness through hard work and diligence. His childhood was certainly not easy, and yet he did not give up because things were hard. He worked and worked to educate himself and make a name for himself when it seems as if the world was against him. August Wilson found his voice through his ability to write. Hopefully, with more research and hard work, kids with apraxia will be able to find their voices, like I have.

(kathy)

A christmas story

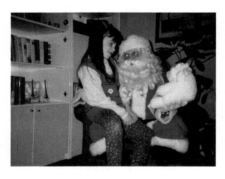

It seems to me that traditions are something that happen slowly and sneak up on you when you least expect it or really have the time for it. At about two and a half years old, Andy's verbal communication skills were non-existent. He had already been in speech therapy for over a year and I had begun to teach him sign language.

When Andy realized that there was a way for him to communicate with me using sign language, he took off. By the time Christmas rolled around in 1996, Andy was four-years-old and using American Sign Language as his primary means of communication. As fast as I could learn it, he had picked it up. He used it every day, with everyone he met, whether they understood or not it didn't matter. He had begun by putting two and three words together and soon after that entire paragraphs, all in sign.

But that Christmas, my concern was Santa Claus. Kate, at seven-years-old was excited and ready for the holiday season. But for the first time, Andy was really aware of what was going on around him at that time of year. It was more than bright lights and yummy smells. It was SANTA CLAUS! And he was ready for it. But I was more than a little nervous. What if Santa didn't understand what Andy was saying? What if Andy finally reached Santa's lap and Santa just didn't get it? I tried to help Andy prepare for this problem by letting him cut pictures of the toys he wanted from catalogues and gluing them to what would become his list. But even still, I worried what if Santa didn't get it?

I decided to make going to see Santa a family outing and got Katie, and Andy, and myself all dressed up. We went to downtown Pittsburgh and took in all the store windows, had lunch and found ourselves in Horne's. This was as good a place as any, I thought, and the line wasn't too long, so we dove in and took our chances.

While we waited in line, both kids practiced what they were going to say. Andy was of course supplementing his grunts with amazingly accurate sign language. As we got closer to Santa, my stomach started to churn. I desperately wanted this to be a good experience, yet I had absolutely no control. What if Santa didn't get it?

Finally, it was our turn. Santa reached out to Andy and took him into his lap. Andy started with the sign language and the paper with the pictures on it. I held my breath. Somehow Santa got it! He signed right back to Andy and used Andy's picture list to find out exactly what this little boy wanted for Christmas. I couldn't help it, I started to cry. He spent the next fifteen minutes with my child and made him feel like the only kid there. And then he did the same with Katie. This department store Santa had made my child feel just like any other kid that went to see Santa. As we were leaving, Santa got up and tapped me on the shoulder and whispered in my ear, "You're doing a good job, Mom." All the way home, I couldn't stop talking about this wonderful Santa. Katie and Andy couldn't figure out what the big deal was. Wasn't Santa supposed to be all things that are good?

When I got home I immediately called Horne's to tell them how lucky they were to have this man and how lucky we felt to have found him. In my haste to thank them, I forgot to get his name.

A tradition had been born and we loved it because it was completely ours and fit us like a tradition should. The next year we did everything just the same-got all dressed up and traveled to downtown Pittsburgh. We looked in all the store windows and had lunch and headed to Horne's to our Santa's lap-only to find Horne's had discontinued Santa. They were closing the downtown store. I guess it was no longer profitable to have Santa on the Christmas floor. We simply returned home. I had no idea what to do next.

I tried to tell myself that this was just a Santa. I couldn't get this upset about a department store Santa, but I knew in my heart that this man, whoever he was, was much more than "just" a Santa. I even took the kids to see the Santa at the mall, but still, I had a mission. I had to find this guy. I just had to.

The first thing I did was call Horne's at South Hills Village near our house. I got connected with a woman named Alex. I told her the whole story. She knew exactly who I was talking about, but no, she didn't know his name. She did, however, have a friend who worked for the management company at Station Square and she thought Station Square might have our Santa. My next call was to Diane at Station Square. Yes, they had tried to get him but no, they hadn't succeeded. But, she did know his name. Unfortunately, Diane didn't feel comfortable giving out his name over the phone. So I gave her my name and number and asked her to have him call me if that was at all possible. It was now December 20th and my children hadn't seen our Santa yet.

I didn't have to wait long before Wayne Brinda called and introduced himself. It was our Santa, on our phone, and I had found him. That was the good news; the bad news was that this was his last day at the Downtown Kaufmann's where he had been all along. I was truly upset; to have gone this far and to have finally found Wayne, only to miss him by hours. I thought about going and getting the kids out of school, but we still couldn't have made it in time. Then Wayne suggested that maybe he could come to our house, although he'd have to check with Kaufmann's to see if he could borrow the suit. He'd call back.

I waited and waited, finally Wayne called back. It was all set, he and his wife Connie would come to our house on Monday, December 23. I was like a little kid myself. I had a secret and my kids were in for a big surprise.

Dinner Monday night was excruciating. Finally, I finished with the dishes. When the appointed hour came along and the doorbell rang I let Katie and Andy open the door, and standing there was our Santa. He was so amazing. He sat with Andy in our big comfy chair for almost an hour. He never forgot Katie and made her feel special too. I couldn't stop crying and tried to hide behind the video camera. He made communication with Andy seem effortless, even though Andy was so excited that any speech skills he had were forgotten. Santa asked each child what was one special thing they really wanted for Christmas. Both kids decided that Beanie Babies were the one thing they had to have for Christmas. Santa promised them Beanie Babies. Then he was gone!

I was trying to figure out where we were going to get Beanie Babies the day before Christmas when the phone rang later that night. It was Wayne and he wanted to thank me for the opportunity to get to know my children. I started to cry some more! This incredible man was so generous and here he was thanking me.

However, the Beanie Baby situation still remained. Christmas Eve day found me on the mad Beanie Baby search. My Christmas shopping had been done since early in November, but here I was with the late crowd counting down the hours. However, after finding our Santa, no mission was too big and Beanie Babies were soon wrapped and waiting under the tree.

You would think that was the end of the story, but then again you don't know Wayne. When I opened the door the next morning, there on the front porch, waiting patiently to be found, were the Beanie Babies Santa had promised. I was totally overwhelmed by this man's kindness and generosity of spirit. He was truly Santa Claus-our Santa Claus.

In my search for Santa, I found him in friends and neighbors and strangers I had never met before, but most surprising, I found him here in my very own home. So when my children ask me, and they inevitably will, if there really is a Santa, I will have to be honest with them and say yes and I have had the real pleasure of knowing him.

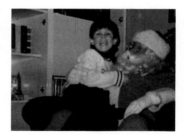

That's not the way I remember it!

Every story has two sides to it and that has always fascinated me. A person could grow up his or her entire life thinking something happened a certain way, only to one day 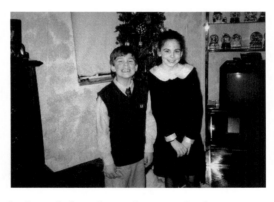 find out the incident had a whole other side to it. And once you have the bigger picture, the whole story changes.

I am of course talking about myself and something that happened when I was a kid and the truth of the story that I found out as a teenager. For as long as I could remember, Andy and I would go see Santa Claus in one of the department stores in downtown Pittsburgh. I remember this so clearly, not because I loved the sights and sounds of Christmas, but because it was the time of year that I dreaded with every fiber of my being. Dreading the family excursion to see Santa wasn't so much about dear ol' Saint Nick, but it had everything to do with my not-so-sweet ol' Mom.

Every year at Christmas, Mom would dress me up and I'm not just talking about wearing a pair of patent leather shoes to town. That was every other day of the year. On this special day that included a picture with Santa, she really outdid herself, complete with big foo-foo dresses and heaven-forbid, THE COATS! Oh, the coats.

There were two coats that just cling to my memory and thoughts of which sometimes still wake me up at night; one was navy blue and one forest green, and the sheer amount of padding in these things had to be enough to insulate a four-bedroom house! Not only did they make me look ten times my actual size, but these coats made me feel as if I was the girl in *Willy Wonka and the Chocolate Factory* that swelled up and turned blue, especially if I was forced into the blue one. After being packed into one those coats, seeing Santa didn't seem so bad.

I remember having to wait in line and watching all the little decorations that the workers had set up, glittering and twinkling, all the while having to patiently wait my turn with my brother to see Santa. We would wait and wait and finally we would be next in line. Waiting was always the most agonizing part, being close enough to watch him interact with some other little kid and not be able to run to him. I remember how Andy would get so excited that he could barely control his delight. I could always tell that my mom was caught in the middle of having to decide to either try to calm him down or just let him go all out. Usually, she chose the latter.

But just like most childhood stories, this one had another side to it. My mom apparently was always inwardly concerned about us seeing Santa. When you have someone in your family with childhood apraxia of speech, things that are everyday occurrences for other families are moments for you that aren't very normal at all. My mom evidently worried that Andy and I would not get to experience these normal things in the same way that all the other kids would. Going to see Santa Claus was something my mom worried about. She wanted us to have the chance to go and meet Santa Claus just like every other child, but she was concerned about how we would be able to communicate with him. Only a mom would ever think this much about what is essentially an everyday activity, but that's what happens when your kids can't talk. And just like a lot of other stories about Andy and I growing up, my mom and I have two entirely differing points of view.

To her, going to see Santa was terrifying because she didn't know if either one of us would be able to properly communicate in a way that Santa would be able to understand. To me, going to see Santa was always a kind of "grin-and-bear-it" sort of thing. Apart from those *delightful* articles of clothing, I never looked forward to actually sitting in Santa's lap. I was always afraid of sitting down too hard and causing his entire leg to fall off. Imagine how many kids would despise me then! Andy, on the other hand, usually flung his entire body on top of Santa's lap with an enormous smile from ear to ear.

Even though my mom was worried about how the speech thing would go, Andy and I never connected Santa Claus with our inability to communicate like other children. And yet, ten years later, I have conversations with my mom and realize there was a whole other side to most of the everyday things that Andy and I took for granted. Not once in all those years did I ever think of not being able to tell Santa what I wanted for Christmas; not once, not ever. It just wasn't two things that I connected. That is until I had a conversation with my mom a couple of months ago. She started talking about how she was always so worried about Santa and our ability to communicate and I just stood there with a dumbfounded expression on my face. I had no idea.

"What are you *talking* about, Mom?," I asked her thinking this time she had gone completely around the bend. And from there, she started talking about how speech had *always* played a role in going to see Santa. And right there, I think I finally got it. I finally comprehended that having a child with childhood apraxia of speech changes *everything*, even the mundane things you would never think twice about, like Santa.

That first year we went to go see Santa is pretty blurry. I vaguely remember Andy signing to Santa Claus and Santa signing right back. I thought that was beyond cool because I had never heard of anything like that actually happening, not even in the movies. But then again, he was Santa, he could do everything! I distantly remember all this. It's the years following that have become the lasting memories.

I was in first grade. At that time the whole hand clapping, rhyming game thing was pretty big at my school. We were always clapping on the playground. One game in particular had become pretty popular in our school. You would tell someone to give you a high five in the air, then down low, then you would say some sort of "witty" remark and then your hand would be in the other person's face. Confused? It was weird, but it was the "big thing" at the time. So of course, that holiday season I decided to test out my new hand clapping skills on Santa. He grinned like any adult would, knowing full well that it was pretty obnoxious and, needless to say, my mother was glaring at me from the other side of Santa's throne. When we got to the car, she definitely let me know what she thought of the whole "hand clapping game." I felt bad that I had done that to Santa.

A couple of days later we were playing a board game after dinner in our living room when the doorbell rang. I should have known something was up though because we never played board games on week nights after dinner, especially in the living room. My mom let my brother answer the door, and once again, looking back I should have instantly become curious because my mom never let either of us kids answer the door, ever! So, Andy goes to open the door, and right there, *in our doorway*, is Santa Claus! I was a seven-year-old, just on the verge of no longer believing in Santa, only to find him knocking at my door.

I remember this night so vividly because nothing, absolutely NOTHING, like this had ever happened to us! I remember Andy sitting in Santa's lap mixing his signing and actual words this time, talking to Santa, and I just stood there with a grin on my face. Then Mom comes behind me and whispers into my ear, "Guess this is your second chance, kiddo!" And I stood there for a second; thinking for just a moment, before an enormous grin spread over my face. I had felt pretty guilty for playing that stupid prank on Santa only a few days ago, and so to have this second chance to make up for it was really special.

When Santa asked, both Andy and I told Santa that the one thing we really wanted was Beanie Babies! We chatted with Santa's "elf" who was rather tall and blonde for an elf. At the end of our visit we walked Santa to the porch and he began to tell this story of how his reindeer were afraid of humans, so they preferred to stay in the sky away from the people while Santa was delivering his gifts. But once night fell and the sky was dark and all the humans went to bed, the reindeers would be okay with coming down and eating some very special 'reindeer mix.' Andy and I sprinkled the reindeer mix that Santa had brought all over our front yard. I would just like to quickly note for the record that according to my mom, that "reindeer mix" was oatmeal with glitter. That's right-apparently reindeer mix doesn't really exist!

That night was so remarkable, astonishing, and enchanting, even if the reindeer mix was just oatmeal. Santa had come to our house, *our house,* and not the mall. But what really got Andy and me thrilled beyond belief was the next morning. We had spent the morning opening tons of presents. There were loads of Beanie Babies situated very nicely on top of our gifts. When my mom opened the door to get the newspaper, she quickly yelled for us to come to the front door. There on the porch were yellow ducks, Beanie Baby yellow ducks. We knew it was from Santa, and in that magical Moment, I truly believed in Santa and believed that I always would.

Of course when we returned to school from holiday break, the kids in my class kept talking about how Santa didn't exist and, close your ears, how our parents *actually* bought the presents. I though was adamant, "You're all wrong. Santa is real, and he came to my house!" Of course the annoying boy snickered, "No kidding, he supposedly comes to all of our houses." None of that mattered though, and I kept believing in my special night with Santa.

Though, as the year went on, that Christmas seemed further and further away, and I didn't argue when my classmates talked about how there wasn't really a Santa. I sadly slipped back into believing that there wasn't a Santa. However, once again, Dear Old Saint Brinda came into my life, changed my mind, and I believed again.

Stepping into line, I was rather reluctant to have to see Santa at the mall. I was of course nine years old and having to sit on Santa's lap was not what I thought nine-year-olds should have to do. However, what happened when we stepped into the room and Santa saw both Andy and I changed my mind, again. When Santa saw Andy and me, he smiled with the biggest, happiest smile I'd ever seen and exclaimed: "Katie and Andy! I'm so happy to see you!" I was shocked! Then he asked if we had gotten our Beanie Baby ducks the previous year. I was amazed, but still a little bit hesitant. I was, after all, nine. At the very end, while my mom and Andy started to leave, I stood off to the side for a little bit, waiting for the next family to come into the room, waiting to see if Santa knew their names as well. I thought maybe my mom had somehow whispered our names to Santa, but as I watched the next family step on up, Santa didn't say their names, and so in that moment, I felt pretty darn special.

As the Parent-Teacher Association President of our elementary school, one of my mom's duties was to write a letter for the monthly newsletter. Mom being, well, Mom, loved this job and took this as a chance to release her inner creative bug. Every month she wrote a humorous yet endearing story about some facet of her life. She decided to write the story of our Santa for one of her December newsletters. It wasn't until I stumbled across this newsletter when I was in middle school and no longer believed in Santa Claus that was I finally understood the whole story of our Santa and Mr. Brinda's role in the story.

I was shocked that such a story could occur throughout the years without me picking up on it. It was enchanting to think such a thing could actually happen outside of the movies, and to Andy and me of all people. The thing that really stood out to me, and still does to this day, is what a kind man Wayne Brinda truly is. To think he made house *calls*....IN A SANTA SUIT! It was inspiring to me that a man as delightful and kind as Mr. Brinda, had not only taken the time to come to our house as Santa, but also to make me believe, if only for a little while longer.

I decided that someday I want to meet Wayne Brinda and properly thank him for all that he did for Andy and me. When I told my mom this she was amused. Confused, I asked why she thought it was funny that I wanted to meet this guy, and she replied:

"You've already met him."

"Other than Santa Claus?," I asked.

And she went on to talk about how Andy and I had already met Wayne Brinda on a field trip to our local theater to see <u>The Witch of Blackbird Pond</u> as students in our mom's theater class. Apparently, after Mr. Brinda was our Santa Claus, he and my mom had kept in touch when they discovered they shared a love of theater and that Mr. Brinda was the co-founder and artistic director of the PrimeStage Theatre Company.

I was amazed that I had actually already met this man. Of course I don't remember him as Wayne Brinda, but I'm not sure if that matters. I might not remember what he looked like on that day in the theater, but I do remember what he looked like as my Santa Claus, what his laugh sounded like, and how he had me believing in Santa Claus for a few more years. That's the point of the holidays though, right? Second chances, believing anything is possible, if only for a night. I will hold those memories close to my heart for the rest of my life. Wayne Brinda had the ability to make a potentially complicated, embarrassing, and perhaps even heartbreaking situation into one of the best and more meaningful moments in my entire life. Thank you, Santa.

Insurance:
Who's gonna pay?

I have written a lot about insurance. I have written about how to fight with your insurance company and how to create paper trails that would make any lawyer smile and welcome parents as clients. What I haven't written about is how these companies make you feel and what happens when you hang up the phone.

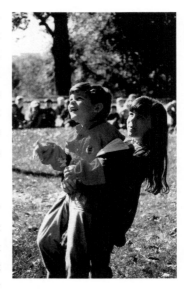

Kate and Andy's apraxia was very different from one another's, but it was obvious from the start that both children would need a great deal of intervention if they had any chance at all of learning to speak effectively. A very conservative estimate of the cost of speech therapy needed before each child started kindergarten was approximately $63,000. That does not account for the four years Katie remained in therapy after she started school or the therapy that Andy continues to receive as he enters middle school.

What I should have done at the very beginning was apply for a medical access card to help defray the cost of speech therapy. MA cards are granted to families based on the disability, not on a family's income. When Kate was six-years-old and Andy was three-years-old my monthly premium for health insurance was greater than my mortgage! I interpreted the health insurance policy handbook to say that the children's speech therapy should be covered. I decided to insist that Blue Cross/Blue Shield stand by their contract and pay for speech therapy for my two children. So began my follies with the insurance companies.

Over the years I have had a number of different health insurance policies. In the early to mid-1990s when the kids first started speech therapy, I had the basic, old fashioned, Blue Cross/Blue Shield health insurance. Everything was fine. It was an 80%-20% split. What that really meant was if the insurance company had an allowable expense of $50 per hour for speech therapy and the therapist charged $100, the insurance company would only pay 80% of $50. So the family would have to pay 20% of $50 and then the remaining $50. Got it? What you really end up being responsible for is $60 and the insurance company pays $40. But still, it was better than nothing.

Next came University Health Network (UHN) in the late 1990s and the first time I would hear the words "medically necessary." Before I switched to UHN, I called the customer service number and tried to make sure that speech therapy for apraxia would be covered. I was assured that all would be well. A few things would be different than the old policy, but the woman on the phone was quite sure that there would be no problem. We would need a new approval every 4 to 6 weeks and because the therapist that we were using was "out of network," the rate of coverage would be less, of course. And the need for the therapy would have to be "medically necessary," of course. But that, I was assured, would not be a problem. Go ahead, I was told, no problem.

Well, that was easy. So easy I never got the woman's name who told me all that. Neither did I get the approval number for the coverage. I didn't even know there was an approval number.

UHN was always behind in making payments to therapists, so it wasn't until almost three months later that I realized that no payments were being made on behalf of my daughter. It was the day before Thanksgiving and I had the flu. I called UHN to try and figure out what the problem was. I tried to be calm. I tried to be nice. I lost my temper. The woman on the other end of the phone informed me that no one was going to bother with all this the day before Thanksgiving and not to bother calling on Friday because it was a holiday and they all had families. Before I hung up on her I gently tried to inform her that I thought the fact that she had children and a family was truly wonderful and I sincerely hoped they would all be healthy and happy over the holidays, because my children never got one second of any day of their lives where they weren't dealing with their disabilities and all that went with it.

Therein lies the whole problem with all of this: the person on the other end of the phone could care less about you and your family. They could care less that you are lying awake at night trying to figure out a way to make all this work. They have a script to follow and quotas to meet and that is that. They don't care what happens when you hang up the phone.

There is so much guilt in dealing with all these insurance issues with regard to your children, too. One phone call can last over an hour because it can take twenty to thirty minutes of beautifully canned music to actually get to a real, live person. It can take many, many calls to "maybe" resolve one problem. In many families, Dad is unavailable to help. He's at work trying to keep his job so that you can keep the insurance coverage that isn't paying for anything anyway. At any rate, Mom is left to make the call and manage the kids at the same time. The TV is the only answer. Plop the kids in front of the TV and hope they don't go blind from sitting too close. As long as you're listening to the lovely, calming music on the other end of the phone, the kids are fine. But the minute you get a real person on the other end all hell breaks loose in the family room and everyone is screaming. When it's all said and done and you've just gone a few rounds with the anonymous voice from the insurance company and you could really use a few minutes of down time, guilt makes you stride into the family room with your most perky voice and say, "Anybody up for Candyland?"

It was after a few months of days like this and denials piled sky high that I decided I couldn't take it any longer and in 1996 I filed a notice of intention to sue Blue Cross and Blue Shield. That one little filing worked so much better than me threatening to go to Oprah all the time. Before anything else of a legal nature could take place, the insurance company paid all of Katie's past therapy bills.

While all this was going on, I had to change insurance companies again. This time it was Select Blue. It might seem like I changed insurance companies all the time, but this was all over a period of years and job changes and it all seemed to make sense at the time. At any rate, I ended up with Select Blue. Every four to six weeks I needed re-approval for each child. Every four to six weeks I put together a packet for each child that included: pregnancy and birth records, letters from all therapists and teachers involved with my children, progress reports and progress notes, and the results of any testing done since the last approval.

At one point, Select Blue decided that Andy's apraxia was no longer severe enough to warrant private speech therapy. They said that I should take advantage of the Early Intervention services that were available. When I called to start the appeal process, the voice on the other end of the phone was astonished that I would even think that Select Blue would give Andy approval for any kind of therapy when I had filed a lawsuit against UHN for Katie several years earlier. Very few times in my life have I been stunned into complete silence, but this was definitely one of them. I gently hung up the phone and called the Pennsylvania state insurance investigator.

By this time, it was a little after five o'clock in the afternoon. With his secretary obviously gone for the day, the gentleman picked up his own phone. By the time my story had tumbled out, I had found an ally. Within 24 hours, Katie and Andy's therapy was not only paid to date, but prepaid for the next three months. It's nice to make new friends.

Needless to say, there was a lot of ranting and raving in my house that night. But when the dust settled, more lawsuits threatened and the bills paid as they should have been by the insurance company, two questions remained: first, does a private company that you pay a premium to every single month have the right to refuse to pay for services because they are also offered through a government program? We were, in fact, already participating in Early Intervention for Andy and the EI therapist had written a letter to our insurance company stating that Andy's issues were so severe that he would benefit from a combination of public and private therapies. I have never heard of such a letter being written for anyone else. The other question that has always bothered me is this: who is the person or committee that is making these decisions on behalf of my children? Are they qualified speech and language pathologists certified by the American Speech-Language-Hearing Association? Have they read the research and are familiar with current thoughts on treatment for apraxia in children? Are they even familiar with speech issues? Have they ever heard of apraxia?

For many years now I have had Preferred Blue. Things have been quiet lately, but those premiums are rivaling the mortgage again. Finally, all the speech therapy bills are paid off. From where I am now, I look back and I can see the emotional cost that was also paid. When we were not at some therapy session and I should have had the time to make a life and memories for my children outside of their disabilities, I was on the phone arguing with the insurance company. Fortunately the kids don't remember it that way, but I do and it still bothers me. The pressure was tremendous. The bills were always getting bigger and there was no end in sight and no one was able to tell me when it might get any easier. Fortunately, the kids' therapist let me pay what I could every month and never even mentioned how huge the balance was getting. But the pressure remained. I struggled through mostly on my own and the cost would turn out to be greater than I could have ever imagined. But today both kids are doing great and I'm still standing.

That insurance thing

One of the topics of conversation that almost always comes up in discussion at CAS conferences is insurance. Ever since that first workshop in Fairfax, Virginia I've been sitting in the back of lecture halls hearing about 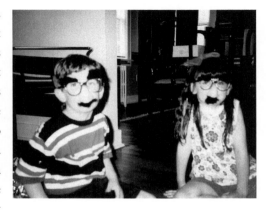 insurance issues as they relate to children with apraxia. This has been a topic of discussion for the past ten years and to be completely honest, I've mostly always ignored it.

Is there anything more boring to a young girl than numbers, and insurance issues and problems? Is there anything more boring at any age than the topic of insurance? Growing up, insurance was always that Blue Cross thing on the plastic card that my mom would have to show the nurse on the way into the emergency room. In all good faith, I cannot portray myself as an expert on insurance. In fact, the thought of discussing my personal life with a stranger on the phone terrifies me. Insurance was never something that was on my radar, until now that is.

A few years ago I started to realize the connection between insurance and the guilt I felt towards my mother. I know that it sounds absurd for me to talk about feeling guilty over having apraxia. Most of the time if there is a conversation about a child with a disability, it revolves around the guilt a parent may feel. Parents will often wonder if they did something to cause their child to have issues or they will feel bad that they can't do more to fix things for their child, but whether my own mother feels this or not, I do.

Before Andy and I were ever blips on my mother's radar, she studied theater at Saint Mary's College in South Bend, Indiana. She flourished and thrived in the theater community and loved every minute of it. In what was once, and perhaps is still, a largely male-dominated field, she studied lighting design. After college, she continued to work in theater, until she became pregnant with me and the word "apraxia" became part of her vocabulary. Gone were the days and nights working on a show. Days were now spent in doctor's offices and the waiting rooms of various speech therapists. Nights were spent reading the latest literature on apraxia and worrying how this was all going to end. Then Andy came along and what was once just one child with a speech disorder suddenly became two children with very complicated disabilities. Her days working in theater must have seemed like someone else's life to my mother. When parents are told that their child has been diagnosed with apraxia, their entire worlds are turned upside down. The future they once envisioned, not just for their children, but also for themselves, is abruptly pulled out from underneath them.

Having a child seems like a pretty expensive proposition: food, diapers, toys, doctor's appointments, clothes, furniture, and so many more things I can't even imagine. It seems positively monumental to think of how expensive a child with apraxia would be; all those sessions of therapy every week that insurance may or may not pay for. Then there are all the other costs that come up: gas, special toys, not to mention time. There are emotional costs that affixing a number to would be impossible. Friends and family who do not understand go by the wayside and parents become isolated. They are thrust into a world they don't understand where speech therapy, and lots of it, is the only way to help their child. At first, parents might think that the health insurance company that charges mighty premiums every month will be their safety net. But it's not too long before they realize that the insurance company is the enemy and is the thing that stands between them and getting the help they need for their child. Yup, you bet there are costs to having a child with a disability.

As someone with resolved apraxia, I do feel guilty that while I was growing up my mother had to cut back on many things in order to find ways to pay the insurance company and all the therapists for my brother and me. I feel awful that there were almost certainly many nights when she cried herself to sleep, utterly petrified, wondering where she would find enough money to pay for all the therapies Andy and I needed.

Over the years, I've had the privilege of meeting so many amazing families from across the world that are going through the same struggles and hardships of raising children with apraxia as my family did. The thing that always stands out to me are the difficulties that occur with families as they try to find ways to pay for therapy. I hear firsthand from these families about how insurance companies will not cover the cost of speech therapy sessions. I don't really understand the problem. Families pay the premiums every month and yet children are still suffering and going without the one thing that would help them: speech therapy. The journey through apraxia is challenging enough without having to fight with your insurance company to pay for what they should be paying for anyway. An insurance company's' bottom line should not be at the heart of a decision on whether to pay for a child's speech therapy or not, but rather the potential of any child should be the driving force behind any decision regarding that child.

I know that I am young and I'm not going to pretend that I understand that much of anything about insurance, but I do wholeheartedly know what it feels like to be a part of a family with a child with disabilities. I do know that a family should be concerned with finding the best ways to support their child, not how they will find the means to finance that support. I've seen how it affected my mother, having to constantly worry about paying for therapy, and my only question is this: doesn't she already have enough to worry about without insurance companies making things all the more difficult? I don't need to fully be able to grasp the numbers and legal issues concerning insurance to realize how wrong it is for companies to be taking advantage of parents who are already dealing with enough.

(kathy)
Conversations with kate

When my daughter, Kate, first started speech therapy at two-and-a-half years old, the therapist recommended that she also start to attend a preschool program. I was, to say the least, resistant to the idea. After all, I was a stay-at-home Mom and 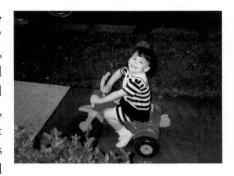 wasn't that what I was there for? But I began to look for preschools anyway. I was in over my head with this apraxia thing and needed some help; so preschool it would be. I interviewed and toured all the schools in the area and for one reason or another, none of them was suitable. Finally, the very last school that I looked at had the most important requirement...I would be allowed to stay until Kate and I felt comfortable being apart.

Kate did great, but she really was unhappy if I tried to leave. A lot of places will tell you just to leave and the child will be fine five minutes after you leave. I guess that's probably true, but I could not leave a child who could not communicate. It just wasn't going to happen. Everyone there seemed fine with that, and I just hung around a few years until they actually hired me!

Kate was finding playmates. She was always a very social child and loved to be in the middle of whatever was going on. But because of her difficulties with communicating, real friends were hard to come by. If Kate was at one end of the spectrum verbally, then her one real friend was at the other. This child was very patient in letting Kate take the time to communicate. I was so happy that Kate had a friend. It meant the world to me.

You think you're going along just fine and everything is going to be okay and then something happens and your world comes crashing down without regard to the tattered mess it leaves behind. That's what happened to me one, bright, beautiful summer day, right in my own back-yard. Kate was about three years old and she had a friend over to play.

Whenever Kate had a play date I was always close by in case she needed an interpreter. The girls were running around the backyard, swinging on the swings, and playing in the sandbox when the little girl wandered over to where I was sitting. "I'm going to be in a wedding," she said. "Wow," I said. "Do you get to wear a fancy dress?" We were off and running having a conversation. Kate rambled over to where the little girl and I were deep in a discussion about weddings.

Kate sat for a few minutes watching us talk, never trying to join in. I didn't really pay any attention to her. I was having fun talking to the little girl. I didn't know you could talk to little girls like that! Kate eventually wandered away and sat in the sandbox, playing by herself. The little girl and I continued to talk about her dress, her hair, the party after the wedding. Later, the child went back to play with Kate and they both were soon building castles in the sand. I sat watching them and it hit me like a ton of bricks. I had never, ever had that *type of conversation with my own child*...that kind of back and forth, give and take. And what's more, I didn't know if I ever would. The fact was that no one in Kate's life, no doctor, no therapist, no one, was able to tell me if Kate would ever be able to communicate with her voice in an intelligible manner. Something broke in me that day. I felt like my heart had been torn away and it was never going to get better. I began to cry and I couldn't stop. Even now, all these years later, when I think of that day, I still can't stop the tears. I can still remember how it feels after all this time.

I felt guilty for enjoying that conversation. I felt guilty for letting Kate just wander away and for not finding a way to include her. I really had no idea what to do or where to turn. You think as a parent you should always have the answer, know what to do, know how to fix things. Apraxia was something that couldn't be "fixed." I had no where to turn and I was pretty sure there really weren't any answers. But being a parent also means not having the luxury of feeling that bad for very long. So I picked my broken self up, pulled myself back together as best I could, and tried to move forward.

Life became a smorgasbord of therapy and we practiced anywhere and everywhere we could. It was always a game, so Kate thought it was fun. Kate never seemed to mind going to "talking practice" as we called it; she liked interacting with adults. If there is any silver lining to all this, it would have to be the ease Kate now has with adults. I can only chalk it up to all those hours of one on one therapy with adults. All total, it was seven long years of therapy for Kate.

Parents will often ask me what the right amount of therapy is for a child with apraxia. Parents with children who suffer want rules. Unfortunately, there really are no rules for apraxia. If your child has appendicitis, you get an appendectomy and everything is okay. Apraxia doesn't work that way. There are no hard and fast rules, no therapy formulas that will make it all better. It all depends on the child, and back in the day, parents had to pretty much figure out what was right for their own child. From the very beginning, though, Kate understood the relationship between talking practice and talking to her friends. There was no such thing as too much therapy in Kate's world. Then Andy came along and I did the same things for him that I had done for her. But Andy had his own little personality and he absolutely did not appreciate overdoses of therapy. At three-years-old he could tolerate a longer session and did much better with speech therapy fewer times a week. It took me a really long time to figure that out. It just depends on your child. He will let you know what's best for him.

I recently asked Kate if she had any memory of what it was like when she was little or of that day by the sandbox. She gave me a funny look and said, "Why would I remember something like that?" She does not remember a time when she could not talk. She does however remember being "dragged" off to speech therapy "all the time." Go figure! That moment in the backyard changed me forever. I would never be that careless again with a child's feelings. I made a promise to myself and to my children that day: whatever I was involved with, on whatever level, I would try to make those around me feel included. Sometimes I am better at keeping my promise than others. But at the end of the day, in that moment between being awake and being asleep, when you have to answer for the day in your heart, it is that promise that guides me.

(kate)
Pretzels and ice cream

I absolutely do not remember that day when my mom and my friend talked about weddings in our backyard. The first time I heard my mom talk about that day in one of the speeches that we gave, I was surprised again at how my memory is so 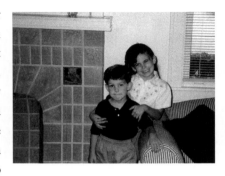 different than my mom's. I grew up in my mother's house and we lived through many of the same things, especially where apraxia is concerned, and yet our recollections are so very different sometimes.

From the vantage point of a young adult, thinking back to that day in my backyard, I can't help but feel a certain amount of guilt. The fact that my mom was so sad because of something as simple as talking with a little girl breaks my heart. Having a conversation with a child is something that is taken for granted in most families, but there was my mom not even knowing that something like that was even possible. Knowing my mom, I can clearly see how she would get caught up in that moment. I can also see her mind processing that children that age could actually talk and she would suddenly understand the depth of the divide between those children and her children.

That day must have been a turning point for my mom. Most people think of getting your driver's license, graduating from high school, going off to college, as the really big moments. But I think that one day, a day that I don't even remember, was a turning point for my mom. It might seem like the days that Andy and I were first diagnosed with CAS might be the really significant days, but this day, this beautiful, calm summer day, that was the day. On that day, she understood fully and completely what having apraxia meant for her children and for herself.

When each of us was diagnosed, my mom was told that we may not ever be able to communicate with our voices, never talk, blah,... blah,...blah. It was that day in my backyard that all those things the doctors had said at the very beginning began to be real, and not just words or predictions anymore. On that day, my mom thought about how she might never have a conversation with either Andy or me, ever. It must have been absolutely terrifying.

I feel bad that my mom had to go through all that, to feel so alone and to be left so in the dark about what the future might hold for her children. It is heartbreaking that she felt guilty in the first place for having a conversation with another child. I wish she could have enjoyed those conversations for what they were and not felt as if she was betraying Andy and me. It's sort of hard to look back on all that and not feel her sadness.

But even though those were apparently some really rough years, neither Andy nor I remember much of the things that made my mom so desolate. At every conference where I speak, there is almost always a parent who wants to know what I think of all the therapy I had when I was younger. The answer is simple: I don't think much of it because I don't really remember much of it. Even though I went to therapy for seven years, the things that I remember are the same things that children without apraxia remember from childhood.

That said, strangely, food is one of the things I do remember most about therapy. At the end of every session we would get these really giant pretzel sticks. I would lick all the salt off the pretzel before I would eat it. I also remember the McDonald's across the street from the therapy office and how we would go there afterwards and get ice cream. Andy and I actually looked forward to those days. The important thing is that these silly little things are what I remember about speech therapy. The therapy itself never really stood out in our lives from my point of view. It did not cast a long shadow on my childhood and it hasn't permanently scarred me as an adult, I think. It was just speech therapy.

My theory is that when people look back on their childhood, they tend to only remember the things that were really momentous, like learning to ride a bike or the first soccer goal. Because therapy blended so naturally into my everyday life, it was never something that stood out from the rest of my childhood, and it certainly never became something that dictated my life outside of the therapy room.

My mom made therapy an everyday thing for both Andy and me. It was never anything special and we were never ashamed of it, mostly because we never really thought twice about it. Every day we practiced our words, our syllables, and our sounds anywhere possible. We would even practice as we went through the grocery store until eventually the people that worked there caught on and helped us practice. We practiced in our car, getting in some last minute repetitions on the way to therapy. Any place you could think of, we've probably practiced speech there. Andy and I never questioned it, it was just the way things were.

Parents worry that the amount of therapy needed when a child has apraxia will cause them to miss out on the rest of their childhood. Andy and I never missed out on anything. We played at friends' houses, we played outside, and we ate lots of ice cream. We did 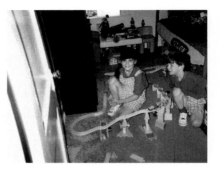 everything all the other kids without apraxia did. We just did something else, too, and I thought of it as fun. My mom always made sure that therapy was something that didn't get us down and because of that, we never felt overwhelmed by speech therapy.

(kathy)
More is not always better!

I was acting like an insane person. Five sessions of speech therapy each week for Katie, five sessions of speech therapy each week for Andy, and one session each week of physical therapy and two sessions of occupational therapy each week for Andy. There was only one day each week where sessions could be scheduled back-to-back to each other. It seemed like we were always in the car, sometimes we even had meals in the car. One thing was certain, we were not going to miss a session of speech therapy or any 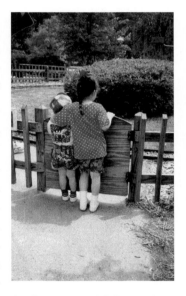 other kind of therapy. I was dizzy with places to be! Then when we were home I was determined that we were all going to have fun, after practicing our speech, of course. It was a totally crazy lifestyle, but I was unwavering in my purpose. These two children were going to be able to speak and speak clearly!

My children are young adults now and they talk beautifully, but I think I was wrong.

It was Andy who taught me that there is a give and take to all of this therapy and he taught me as only Andy can. Kate loved speech therapy and there was no such thing as too much for her. She loved being with adults and seemed to think that speech therapy was really designed as a special time set aside for adults to play with her. She loved to practice her speech at home as it was her time when she had Mommy all to herself. Andy, on the hand, was not so eager or compliant. He had other things on his mind. I remember once when he was in sixth grade we were driving home from school, he was very quiet in the car, lost in thought. I asked him what he was thinking about, fully aware of the dangers of asking a twelve-year-old boy what was rattling around inside his head. "String Theory," he said, "I'm thinking about String Theory." "What the hell is that?," I sputtered. Andy proceeded to elaborate on String Theory and his thoughts and conclusions on the subject. And I had been worried he was going to ask me about girls! But Andy had been like that since he was just a little boy, he was thinking about things that most other kids really didn't even care about. So speech therapy for Andy was an interruption in the things he wanted to think about. He could have cared less if anyone understood his speech, he knew what he was thinking about.

It took me awhile to figure all this out! I had one child with apraxia and I thought that meant I had the whole thing figured out. After all, I had done my homework and I knew what the brightest minds in the world were saying about apraxia. I have to laugh at myself though because when I thought I had it all figured out, the best and brightest minds were still trying to figure out what to call it. It wasn't until 2007 that the American Speech-Language-Hearing Association came out with a position statement that confirmed that apraxia was a disorder found in children. I say, all they had to do was ask me-I knew it was disorder as far back as 1995.

I tried to do the same things with Andy that had appeared to be successful with Kate. What that meant was lots and lots of therapy, at least once a day, followed up by lots and lots of practice at home. Andy also needed physical therapy for the sensory integration disorder that plagued his life. His issues with balance also affected everything from his ability to walk to his inability to ride a bike. Occupational therapy was also a part of Andy's life, as he worked diligently for over a year to learn to tie his shoes. I threw in some equestrian therapy for good measure, mostly because it couldn't hurt and it just might help. I'm exhausted just trying to remember all the therapies that Andy had in his daily schedule. But Andy wasn't buying what I was selling and he hated therapy-any kind of therapy. Andy invented all kinds of distractions: he was a clown, he was too tired, his eyes were everywhere but where they needed to be. Still I plowed on and therapy continued every day. Andy endured, but he wasn't happy. Then came Christmas in 1999, Andy was seven years old and he had had enough.

We love Christmas in our house! The decorations go up right after Thanksgiving and Christmas music blares constantly when we are home. We bake a mountain of cookies and look for secret ways to surprise each other. We love our traditions, but the reality is that it can all be overwhelming, especially if you are little and have issues integrating sensory information and can't communicate. Andy had been working very hard and was making a bit of progress. The speech sounds were coming and we knew we at least had a chance at verbal communication.

I was not always an early riser. As a matter of fact, having spent many years in theater, I was just the opposite, preferring to work late into the night and get up in time for lunch. Of course, having kids changes a person, mostly having children changes the time a person gets up in the morning. On this particularly bright and sunny December morning, I was up and dressed early enough to enjoy my cup of tea before the daily round of visits to various therapists. I was just starting up the stairs to wake the kids when Andy started down the stairs and tripped, falling down the last few. Probably that should have been a clue. But honestly because of Andy's complex series of motor planning difficulties, tripping down the stairs was not the red flag it might have been in another child. The red flag came when Andy tried to say something and nothing came out-nothing at all. It's not an overstatement to say that Andy went to bed one night with the ability to make some speech sounds and even some words and woke up the next morning having lost every single skill he had worked so hard to acquire. "Oh my God, what the heck, what do I do now?," I thought.

Trying hard not to be hysterical, I methodically worked through the sounds and words that I knew Andy could produce. I got nothing but grunts, groans, and a high-pitched screamy kind of noise that did nothing to ease my level of panic. I called the office of Andy's primary speech therapist, she wasn't in yet. Okay, I decided that because I saw this woman every single day of my life and I knew as much about her children as she knew about mine, and because she was the key to my children's ability to communicate, and because I trusted her, it would be fine to call her at home. So, I did.

She was, of course, as gracious as I knew she would be. I explained to her that Andy had woken up that morning having lost any and all progress he had made. I did not have to explain my panic. Although it was pretty infrequent, losing all the sounds like Andy had was apparently not unheard of. She felt that Andy might in fact be feeling overwhelmed by the amount of therapy he was receiving, in addition to the excitement of the holiday season. Instead of rushing to the therapist's office, we took the day off and played all day. As a matter of fact, I called therapy off for everyone until the New Year. That was my wakeup call and the day that I began to understand that "more is not always better." It took about a month, but Andy eventually regained the skills that he had lost and we moved on with therapy. But we moved on with a different attitude and I was never afraid again to back off when it all got to be too much and we felt overwhelmed.

There have been a few times along this journey that I have had one of those aha! moments. Though I don't always like change, those moments usually demand that I modify, alter, and adjust my own thought process and consequently, my actions. In 2004, CASANA had the very first National Conference dedicated to childhood apraxia of speech. Five hundred people from all over the world gathered in Pittsburgh, PA to learn from the most highly regarded professionals in the country. Al Condelucci, Executive Director of United Cerebral Palsy in Pittsburgh, agreed to present a session on "Social Capital." Al is a dynamic speaker and I was excited to be able to offer this session to the families attending the conference. I was really interested in this session personally, but as the conference organizer I knew that I wouldn't have time to sit through the entire session. However, as I was passing through the back of the room making sure that everything was going along smoothly, I paused to listen to what Al was talking about-and those few moments completely changed the way I was doing things.

This was my take-away from my short time listening to Al: raising kids with special needs sometimes means focusing on what our kids can't do in order to help them as much as possible. Through the process of always trying to "fix" our kids we forget to recognize the special things about them that make them individuals.

I am a very social person and to me life is a party waiting to happen. Andy is not. What took me so long to figure out is that Andy is not like me in that way. Katie is and so it was easy for me to figure out what she needed and to head us in that direction. But Andy isn't that way and he was just as happy to hang out on his own or with his family and read a technical journal or play with his LEGOs. In spite of the fact that I kept pushing him, Andy didn't want to be the life of the party. He didn't want a million and two friends. As I stood in the back of the room I felt like Al was talking just to me when he spoke about accepting our kids for who they are and to stop trying to make them into something they aren't and usually don't even want to be.

When I stopped pushing Andy into being something he didn't want to be and started accepting him the way he was, when I started to value what was so special about him, he began to blossom. He began to come out of his shell and value those things in himself. That was the key to Andy, teaching him to value the parts of himself that, while different from his peers, were in fact the most precious parts of Andy. When I changed, Andy changed, and all for the better. To come full circle, Andy was recently part of a teen panel at the 2011 CASANA National Conference and he had the audience of 300 parents and professionals in the palm of his hand. He was articulate and funny, and the life of the party.

Lights, camera, buffy?

I attended a small, private
middle school and high school
in Pittsburgh called Shady Side
Academy. It was a great school
and I loved my time there, but
I never really felt like I truly
belonged. I was different than
my classmates and it took me
a very long time to figure out
why and to feel okay about it.
I was focused and I was driven.
I had no interest in the typical
fluff things that girls my age
were supposed to be thrilled

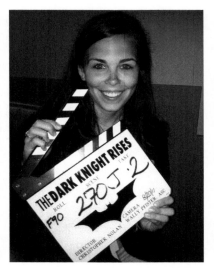

by. Just as my mom had to learn that my apraxia was different than
Andy's and really couldn't be treated in the same way, I had to
learn that my path would be different than my classmates.

For many families at my school, exotic spring break trips were
pretty standard, and kids returned to school after the March break
with stories of skiing in Colorado and laying on the beaches in
the Bahamas. Disneyland was about as exotic as my family got in
those days, but that doesn't mean I didn't go back to school without

exciting stories in March of my freshman year of high school. I had movie cameras following me around that spring. That is definitely an exaggeration, but that's what it felt like and that might be what I told my friends.

My mom had been working on an informational, documentary type of film called *Hope Speaks, An Introduction to Childhood Apraxia of Speech* for the Childhood Apraxia of Speech Association of North America with a Pittsburgh producer/director named Peter Argentine. They had been going around Pittsburgh for a couple of days interviewing parents of children with apraxia, such as Mary Sturm and Sharon Gretz. They were also filming some of the kids around town who had apraxia and it just so happened that I was one of those kids.

At the time I was a fourteen-year-old girl who was set on becoming an actress, so having cameras around seemed pretty awesome to me. My middle school years were pretty typical: drama, obnoxiousness (mostly on my part), and then, more drama. I think the drama at my school was intensified because of how small the school was and how we all lived in each other's back pockets. Television was my escape and when I came home from school each day, it was the show *Buffy the Vampire Slayer* that took me away from all my middle school problems.

I found Buffy in the summer before seventh grade. I was flipping through the channels, came upon Buffy, and I was immediately obsessed. Once school began that year, I enjoyed closing the door on the gossip and scandals of seventh grade and visiting Sunnydale every afternoon.

Until Buffy, I had never really thought about what I wanted to do with my life. The fact that Sarah Michelle Geller playing Buffy could make me feel better about my life made me think that that might be something I would like to do. Could I really help young girls feel better about middle school drama? Could I be an actress?

My interest in the entertainment industry made being involved in *Hope Speaks* the most exciting thing that had ever happened! Even though it was Peter, my mom, and the camera guy who showed up to film my interview, it was an extraordinary experience.

I had a friend over to the house that day because they wanted to film me talking with someone. What that really meant though was that I had to explain apraxia to my friend. It's kind of hard to explain apraxia to someone who isn't a speech language pathologist, but the truth is you have to get used to it because not too many people know what apraxia is. She was the first person outside of my family who I talked to about having the disorder, and thankfully it didn't seem to be a big deal to her.

We shot some scenes with my friend and me eating pizza and dancing to music. It was a bit awkward doing those everyday things with a camera right in the middle of everything, but we both got through it. I also shot a couple scenes on the porch with my mom, and then it was time for my big interview. I was nervous that I would stumble over my words, but it all turned out okay.

Having the chance to witness what it was like behind-the-scenes of making even that small documentary really got me interested in what went on behind the camera. Two years after we shot *Hope Speaks*, I worked as an intern for Peter Argentine. And three years after *Hope Speaks*, I got the chance of a lifetime-the opportunity to work on a full-length feature film.

Before there were movies, though, there was basketball, and soon enough my two worlds would collide. For fifteen years I played basketball. When I was three my neighbor's son, who played basketball for a professional team in Greece, introduced me to the sport that I, too, would come to love. The first basket I ever made, I made from atop his shoulders. From then on it seemed everything in my life revolved around basketball. When I was on the basketball court it never mattered whether my speech was perfect or not as long as I was playing my absolute best. I never missed a game and I never missed a practice.

When I was sixteen, my right kneecap started to slowly dislocate after repeatedly falling on it during the season. I didn't know what the problem was and I didn't tell anyone until I could barely walk. I spent six months trying to rehabilitate the knee, and then had to have the surgery to secure the tendons and ligaments around my knee anyway. I lost the whole year. As I began my senior year, the same thing began to happen to my left kneecap. I struggled through my senior year, but I knew I was done and my dream of playing basketball in college would have to give way to some other dream.

During the three weeks I was bedridden after my knee surgery, I discovered video editing. I loved the way that I could tell different stories just by the way I edited a video. Though my interest in film began with my obsession with *Buffy* and was sparked more with *Hope Speaks*, it also got me through that difficult time when I was reevaluating everything that was important to me. The funny thing was that as I was reassessing what the future might hold for me and looking toward the film industry, it never once occurred to me that I should take the fact that I had apraxia into consideration.

During my senior year of high school, a Lifetime movie came to our campus to shoot a few scenes. From the moment I found out about the movie, I knew I had to be involved. I worked the phones calling everyone I knew and then calling everyone they knew. Finally someone was willing to take a chance on me and I went to work for one day on my first feature film. I ended up directing traffic a half mile away from all the action. I simply didn't care. It was a start.

The production company asked me to stay on the film and work through the weekend and that was when basketball and film came crashing together; and one would have to give way to the other. By this time I understood that playing basketball in college would no longer be an option. I also understood that I was with a group of people who had accepted me and who could teach me so much about making movies. I chose the movie and that was probably the best decision I had made up to that point in my life.

From that day forward I worked pretty steady on local films whenever I wasn't at school. In addition to *Homecoming*, the movie that was filmed at my high school, I have had the amazing opportunity to work on a number of feature films including, *My Bloody Valentine 3D, Warrior, I Am Number Four, Abduction, The Next Three Days, One for the Money, The Perks of Being a Wallflower,* and *The Dark Knight Rises*.

The remarkable thing is that not one of the people I work with now realizes that I had a severe speech disorder as a young child. And while I have no problem telling people about my apraxia, it just isn't something that comes up in conversation very often. In a strange way it really was my apraxia that has led me here, but instead of dictating what I couldn't do, it introduced me to something I could do. I'm excited to see what the future holds, but I know I will always look back to *Buffy* and *Hope Speaks* and know those are my roots.

Why won't my family accept what's going on?

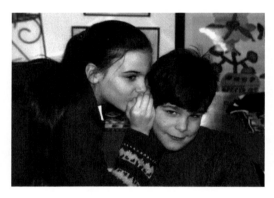

I remember one time, when both my of kids were still toddlers, my mother and I were in downtown Pittsburgh shopping. We got on an elevator with another older woman. She began to talk to my son who could only respond to her with grunts. She asked about his speech and I went into my usual explanation about apraxia that I always used when strangers were kind enough to ask and not just stare. She became a little agitated and shot me down with, "That's just a little speech problem, for heaven's sake!" My eyes began to tear up. How could this woman who knew nothing about my child, myself, or his diagnosis be so judgmental? Thank God my mother understood or I would have been very alone indeed.

I have two sisters and a brother and none of them would be able to dredge up the word apraxia. It's not that they haven't heard it or that I haven't tried to share with them what's going on in my family, it's just not that important to them. Another family member once told me that there was no such thing as apraxia and that the doctors were just taking me for a ride to collect insurance money. I'm pretty sure she might have had apraxia herself, but whatever. I never really expected much, I guess. At the beginning I had high expectations regarding my family. I thought they would sustain me and help me navigate the path we were on. It soon became evident that that my family could not or would not be there for me or my children in the ways that I needed them to be. There was a time though that I had higher expectations.

Katie was born in 1989. In 1991, I was forced to file personal bankruptcy. Katie was diagnosed as developmentally delayed late in 1991, and in 1992 Andy was born. He was put into speech therapy without a diagnosis in 1994 and diagnosed with CAS in 1995. I could have used a little support. It was a lonely time for me.

Mostly, my sisters and brother never acknowledged that my children weren't like other children, like their children. When I tried to talk to them about it, I was met with silence or a quick change of subject. My oldest sister seemed more open to discussion, but my tears were always answered with "everything will be fine." My family isn't big on high emotion. Unfortunately, it's the only way I know how to function. I realize that people say "everything will be fine" in an effort to try to make you feel better or they say that when they have nothing else to say or don't know what to say, but after a while you just want to strangle the next person who says it! When you attend countless sessions of therapy each week, deal with the insurance company, and are trying desperately to give your kids some kind of memories other than therapy, you just don't want to hear that "everything will fine!" You don't want to hear it because you don't believe it. You want, you need, a shoulder to cry on. You need someone to acknowledge your fear that everything might not be "just fine." You need someone to say out loud that they will stand by you every step of the way, no matter where the journey may lead. You need someone to understand just how hard you are fighting this battle and just how battle-weary you really are. I thought that kind of support would come from family.

I have met some families where dealing with one child's diagnosis of apraxia becomes the mission of the entire family. Grandmas go online and deal with the computer beast in order to get information. Aunts and uncles call anywhere they can think of to talk to someone who might know something. I am in awe of these families. And yet, I have also heard from folks who wish their parents and siblings would interfere just a little less. Frankly, I don't get that-good Lord give me some help!

Then there are friends. What can you say about well meaning neighbors and friends who constantly remind you that Einstein didn't talk until he was four and he turned out just fine. As your friends revel in each step their child takes, in each sound that comes out of their mouths, how can you not help but feel sad? It takes a mighty friend to understand that although you are happy that his or her child is talking in sentences at two, you can barely stand to be near that child without bursting into tears. I have found that when I have tried to explain some of my fears for my children to family or friends, they often reply that all parents worry about their children. It is difficult to explain to parents of typical children that while all parents do worry about their kids, what we are concerned about is quite different. One woman I know worries that the gifted program in our school district is not quite up to snuff to suit the needs of her children. And while I understand that this is a real issue, I am worrying whether some young lady will ever see past my son's disabilities and want to make a life with him. I am wondering if he'll ever have a friend to call his own. I am wondering if he will be assaulted in school again this year. Oh yes, I also believe my son may be gifted, but there really is no test that would show that, notwithstanding his disability, so the gifted program in our school district isn't even an option for him.

I think I have met maybe two people who don't have children with disabilities that actually "get it." They also happen to be married to each other. As for the rest of the world, even my pediatrician doesn't really understand. I believe he is a good man and certainly means no harm, but it's painful to have explain what apraxia is every single time I go into his office. Is it any wonder that as a parent you begin to think that no one really cares?

When both my of kids were toddlers, I felt this burden much greater than I do now. I remember thinking that it was so odd that I was the only person who really knew everything that was going on with these kids. I was my family's social worker, which is fine, except I'm a theater major for heaven's sake! What the heck do I know about dealing with kids with disabilities? After all these years of in-the-trenches experiences, I am now confident enough to go the distance, but back then I felt a tremendous weight on my shoulders. I felt like if I made the wrong decision, it would affect their entire lives. I felt like if I made the wrong choice, they may never be able to communicate with their voices. Speech five times a week or four? How much OT? How much PT? Should we get another evaluation? Is she ready for kindergarten or would one more year of preschool give her the edge she may need? Will she ever say blue and not ba-lu? CER, IEP, ADHD, OCD, IFSP, AAC, DAS or CAS, EI, ESY, (sorry you don't qualify), MRI, SID, PECS or ASL, SPED (I never thought it could happen to my child)-it's enough to make a sane girl nuts!

We actually did a have a social worker once. When we used our county's Early Intervention services, she came out to the house once a month or so. Because I served her Danish pastries and coffee when she came to visit, she figured I had everything else under control, too.

I used to know a woman who had a child with Down's syndrome. He was the sweetest, cutest little guy you would ever want to meet. His mom had a tremendous amount of support from family, friends, and agencies. Her husband always bought her the greatest jewelry, for no reason. I used to wonder sometimes, if I couldn't get any help because my kids didn't look disabled. In fact, it was quite the opposite. Both my kids were quite tall for their ages and incredibly cute. It almost seemed as if the bar was raised higher for them and folks expected more mature behavior than they could have possibly produced, especially speech.

The grocery store always seems to bring out the worst in everyone. Our grocery store has a great program, once a year you pay a dollar for a "cookie card." Then throughout the year, each time you visit the store you can go to the cookie counter and ask for a cookie. It's a great bribe to get your kids through the store because the cookie counter is the last stop and stopping is completely dependant on behavior. It was the asking for the cookie that always presented a problem for us. Instead of just telling the lady what cookies my kids wanted, I always let the kids ask for themselves. Of course, it was never that simple. The kids would make some attempt at speech, the lady wouldn't understand, she would make some comment about big kids like them not being able to talk, yadda, yadda, yadda. It was always the same and I would walk away feeling really, really bad. I finally took the bull by the horns and one day explained to the cookie lady all about apraxia and my children's struggles to learn to speak. She became one of our greatest allies. She even learned some sign language as time went on and doled out extra cookies for Mom. Having the cookie lady on your side is not a bad thing, not a bad thing at all.

On some level, the kids I were used to encountering a degree of discrimination and rudeness from some people, but the "Mommy and Me" class that Andy and I were enrolled in still sticks out as one of the most inexplicable examples of bad behavior from an adult dealing with a child's disability that I have ever seen.

Andy was just two, so of course, it all pretty much went over his head. At this point, I knew Andy had some issues, but it would be years before it was all defined and laid out. For now, it was just "Mommy and Me." The teacher in the class was great and there was just enough structure for two year olds. Snack time was always a riot. The kids would all sit at a little table and eat whatever was in front of someone else. One day Andy was sitting next to a child whose mother came off as fairly perfect. She would show up for class in black leather pants and really cool black leather boots; not exactly the best thing for finger-painting, but cool nonetheless. On this particular day, her son grabbed some food out of Andy's hand. Mrs. Perfect rushed over took the food out of her child's hand, gave it back to Andy and said, "Don't take his food son, you don't know if what he has is catchy!!!" I swear I am not making this up! I was completely devastated and so was the teacher. She called me that night and apologized and offered to put us in her other class. I thought we were more tolerant and educated in the 1990s, but I guess I was wrong.

Another woman in that very same class berated me for using sign language with my child when he clearly wasn't deaf! Those of you who have been dealing with apraxia for any amount of time realize that sign language is a tool, just one of many, that we have available to us in dealing with this disability. Sign language gives our children the ability to communicate with their hands until they learn to use their voices. One of the most important things in a child's life is to be able to communicate his wants and needs to those who care for him. Sign language relieves their frustration and gives children with apraxia the ability to do just that. It is also part of that Total Communication package. If a child can see the word and hear the word, he is more likely to say the word. That's the theory. Some parents and clinicians fear that the child will use sign language as a crutch and never attempt speech. I have never been able to find any research that indicates that is true. In fact, when a child is able to vocalize even an approximation of a word, she or he immediately drops the sign. These children want to speak, they are trying to speak, they just need help. Anyway, in retrospect I think I should have just dropped that class.

I was not a very good friend to other adults when my kids were younger. It took days to return calls. I couldn't go out, as babysitters for two children with special needs were few and far between. It is easy to feel isolated. Depression is never far away. As a parent of children with special needs it is almost essential that you develop a kind of tunnel vision. You are learning a new language that includes a lot of medical terms and insurance terms. You must focus on what your child cannot do, in order to help him turn it into something he can do. Joy is found and measured in tiny steps forward, in accomplishments that other parents take for granted. Friends, as well meaning as they may be, can not possibly understand what it is like to sob in the shower because it is the only place that is safe to let your emotions go.

Which brings us back to family. I believe with all my heart that it is your family that should be your foundation and support. They should be ones that understand and keep you going when you think you have nothing left to give your children. They should be there when Mrs. Perfect has ripped your world apart. They should be there when strangers stare and the cookie lady is mean. They should understand that your child making the "ka" sound for the first time is a home run and is cause for celebration. But some of us, a lot of us, actually, are not lucky enough to have those kinds of extended families and so we have to learn to depend on ourselves. If we are really lucky, we can find another parent who has a child like ours or a therapist who becomes a friend. My advice is to find someone. This is a difficult road to travel alone.

I was very lucky in that my mother has always stood right beside us. I think in the beginning it might have been hard for her to really understand all that we were going through. I remember one year we were at the CASANA National Conference in Williamsburg, VA, it was late at night, and we were all lounging in the hotel room, relaxing and chatting. Kate, who by then was in high school, started to talk about how hard it was for her to talk when she was tired. She spoke about the effort that it took sometimes to make everything in her mouth work right. My mother says that was the first time that she truly, truly understood how hard it had been, and still was sometimes, for my kids. Regardless, before and after that my mom has been my sounding board, my rock when I needed her to be, and always, my best friend.

In my family, relationships have become difficult and strained, and some even non-existent. This has been my choice. I found it very difficult to pretend that everything was okay just to make everyone else feel better. In the spring of 2001 I was burning the candle at both ends, as my grandmother used to say, and I ended up extremely ill. I wish I could say that my family came through and I was completely wrong about all of this, but the sad fact is, my illness was off the radar and barely ever mentioned. I have been forced to come to the conclusion that, in my family, if you don't talk about it, it doesn't have to exist and bother you. That's what happened with the kids. If we didn't talk about it, then maybe we could pretend they were just like all the other kids in our extended family. I made the painful decision that I couldn't live that way. It wasn't fair to my children. I have always been up-front and honest with the kids about what their issues are. They have a name for what makes things difficult for them: apraxia. It is a part of who they are and always will be. It has to be acknowledged by those who say they love them. So the end result is that I do not have relationships with the people that I love. I do not have relationships with the people that I want to support in good times and in bad. I can't do it. I have other mountains to climb.

My CASANA family

It's easy to feel alone. It's easy to think that there is no one who truly understands the battles you wage every day against apraxia. Apraxia changes your life in ways that you could

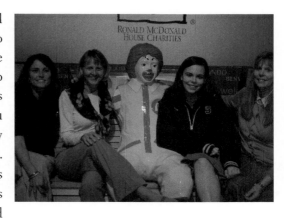

never imagine at the beginning of the journey. Sometimes, your extended family will rise and be there with you every step of the way. And sometimes they won't. When that happens, there are people ready to step in, eager to meet you and share your journey; that is your CASANA family.

I cannot even begin to describe how grateful I am for my CASANA family. In middle school and high school, I traveled to many of the workshops that CASANA held around the country and slowly I built relationships with the speakers and the volunteers. They became the aunts and uncles I hadn't had in my life for so long.

While I was at Saint Mary's College in South Bend, Indiana, my mom earned a reputation for the awesome care packages she would send me. They were filled with all of my favorite things and it was her way of letting me know that she was thinking of me. When my mom was going through some financial hard times, it was Kathy Jakielski who stepped in and made sure that I still had care packages filled with yummy treats and funny presents. Kathy J.'s husband, Dave, is a Notre Dame alum, and every fall I would look forward to tailgating with them and their friends. It was confusing to my friends, though, why my aunt was named Kathy when my mom was also named Kathy.

In the summer of 2011, I finally got to meet Kathy J. and Dave's son Byron at CASANA's National Conference. Byron is a few years younger than me, but still, we hit it off immediately. We are both athletic, though he is the better athlete by far. I remember walking through the halls of the conference center hearing beautiful piano music and wondering why my mother would hire a professional piano player for the event. Turns out it was Byron; in addition to being a high caliber athlete, he is also a gifted musician.

CASANA's 2012 National Conference was held in Boston and we were all there again. Andy, Grams, Aunt Kathy J., and Byron; we took a side trip to Salem and ended up having our fortunes told. Our psychic took us in two at a time and Byron and I went in together to take a peek into the future. The woman immediately said she sensed a strong bond between us and asked how we were related. We paused and looked at each other, before smiling, and replying in unison said, "Cousins." It was a great moment because both of us suddenly realized that it doesn't matter that we have no blood in common; we are family.

Kathy J. is the aunt that was missing from of my life for so long. She is the most generous person I have ever met. She is generous with her heart and she is always there for the people that she loves, including two random kids in Pittsburgh. When Andy graduated from high school it was just going be me, Mom, and Grams there for him. Somehow Kathy J. got wind of this and flew halfway across the country to be there for Andy on his big day. It shouldn't have come as any surprise to me then, that as I was walked down the aisle at my college graduation, standing right there next to my mom was none other than Aunt Kathy J. and Uncle Dave. It wouldn't have felt right if they weren't there.

My CASANA family also came to include Jeanne Lippert or Aunt Jeanne as she has come to be known. I met Jeanne and her husband Kurt in the summer of 2006 when the CASANA National Conference was in St. Paul, Minnesota. Each year, somewhere in the country, there is a family that says "yes" when my mom asks if she can ship the materials for the CASANA National Conference to them. Little do they know that can sometimes mean up to 100 boxes! In 2006, that family was the Lipperts and that is how I met Jeanne and Kurt. After that, Jeanne would at times travel with my mom to help out at workshops. It didn't take long for me to come to love Aunt Jeanne.

In 2008 the CASANA National Conference was held in Williamsburg, Virginia and Jeanne brought her daughter to volunteer at the Conference. Lauren was around 10 years old at the time and I instantly adored her. We hung out, watched movies, and explored Williamsburg-and Lauren became part of our family. We started to call Lauren Little J because she was a miniature version of Jeanne. At this point, Little J comes to the Conference every summer to run the Sales Desk with her mom and I don't think people realize her name isn't LJ. If Byron is my cousin, then Little J is my kid sister.

The summer the National Conference was in San Diego, California, we realized that we had really become a family. There were the aunts:

Kathy J., Jeanne, and my mom; the cousins: Andy, Byron, Lauren, and myself; and, of course, the family matriarch: Grams. The cousins always nag the aunts about getting together for holidays. The family that we created is the family that I love.

I feel like I am truly blessed. The CASANA board members have been there watching over me since I was a child, especially Mary Sturm, M.D., who is always on speed dial for trips the emergency room. Sharon Gretz and her son Luke have been with us for most of our journey with apraxia and have stood beside us through everything.

 While I may not have the actual extended family that should have been there, I have been so lucky to have adopted aunts and uncles and cousins who I get to spend time with every summer. My CASANA family has touched my heart. They have been there for my family time and time again when there was no one else. They are everything to me. It's not Thanksgiving or Christmas that I look forward to each year-it's the National Conference, my family reunion, that I look forward to each summer.

I know it's hard for Mom at times not having the family that she was born with there for her. I know she misses having the people who have known her the longest in her life. But Grams is always there and we have surrounded ourselves with the best family anyone could ever wish for. At the end of the day, the journey through apraxia doesn't have to take things away from your life, it gave us our family.

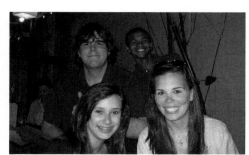

(kathy)

School:
To label or not to label

By the time Katie entered kindergarten, her file was already inches thick! She had been in private therapy, as well as therapy through the Allegheny County Intermediate Unit, for a little over three 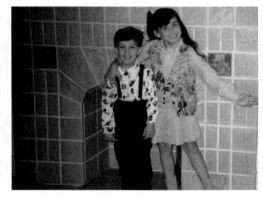 years. There are 29 Intermediate Units in Pennsylvania, formed in 1970 by the PA Department of Education. The AIU is an educational service agency that offers, among many other services, various types of interventions for children with special needs. The AIU is set up a little different these days, but when Kate was younger they offered services to the kids until they entered kindergarten. They also housed most of Kate's files that contained evaluations, progress reports, etc. Some of her files were with her private therapist, copies of almost everything were stored in a third floor closet in my home.

With the combination of therapies, Kate was making tremendous progress, but it was clear that the work was not yet done. I began preparing the school that would become her elementary home school almost a year before Katie would step through the front door.

When I first contacted the school's speech-language pathologist, I don't think she took me very seriously. My problem is that I'm not very good with buzz words. I just can't seem to remember them or put them in the right place in a sentence. I am also not that great on-the-spot. I'm one of those people that has the perfect come back three hours after it's needed. But by our third phone call, I must've used some of the right words, one of which was probably apraxia, because I was soon trying to deal with the mountains of paperwork a transition brings into your life.

One of the decisions that had to be made along the way was whether to "red flag" Katie's files from the Intermediate Unit. This would mean the Intermediate Unit would not pass Katie's information along to the school district. This can be a real double-edged sword for parents. On the one hand, you want the special education folks at the new school to know as much as they can about your child so that they can receive appropriate services as quickly as possible when the new school year begins. On the other hand, some of the stuff in these files can be real nonsense and you don't want your child's new school and teacher to be influenced negatively toward your child. Back and forth I went. On any given day I could argue either side of the debate.

Finally, I called the principal at what would be Kate's new home school. I was curious as to what his thoughts would be on the subject. I carefully explained my thoughts, not wanting to insult the public school bureaucracy or step on any as of yet unknown toes. Finally the good principal gently laughed and said that we would be lucky if anybody actually ever read Kate's file. His problem was getting teachers to even look at the special education files, not keeping the information in perspective. "Ah geez," I thought, not knowing if that was a good thing or a bad thing.

At the end of the day, I came up with what I thought would be the perfect compromise. I would red flag Kate's files from the Intermediate Unit. However, I would let the Special Education Director of the School District have the files for one week to look through and come up with suggestions as to the course of Katie's therapy beginning in kindergarten. A couple years later I was sitting in an IEP meeting, when a piece of paper floated across the table at me from Katie's AIU file. "Where did you get this?" I asked the therapist. It came to light in that meeting that the Special Education Director had in fact copied the AIU file during the week that it had been in her possession. Kate's red flagged AIU file had been part of her elementary school file from day one. All that angst for nothing.

Somewhere between Katie and Andy the rules changed and the AIU turned over responsibility for a preschool-aged child's intervention to the school district when the child turned three years old, although the AIU still provided the actual services. This made the issue of records a moot point and Andy's records were automatically turned over to the school district.

The other worry I had in elementary school was the amount of time each of the kids spent outside the classroom. I believed that three or four sessions of therapy a week were necessary for the kids to make progress with their speech. But if I was able to secure those sessions for each child then that was three or four times per week that the kids were outside the classroom, not learning. That was also three or four times per week that kids had to get up and leave the classroom, drawing attention to the fact that they were leaving and doing something different.

I was always concerned that they would fall behind in class with the amount of time they spent outside of class, especially Andy who also had to fit physical therapy and occupational therapy into his school day schedule. It came down to making up for lost class time at home, carefully going over homework and filling in the blanks from missed classroom time as they came up.

The other issue, worrying about their peers noticing them leaving the classroom, seemed to be more mine than theirs. The reality of our public school system is that kids are coming and going from classrooms all day long. It's no big deal. The kids don't really know where the other kids are going and it could just as easily be a gifted program, or a music lesson, or a speech therapy class. Because of this level of acceptance among the kids themselves, the child leaving the classroom isn't put under a microscope and doesn't feel funny about the fact that he is leaving.

When it was time to think about sending Andy to kindergarten, a few things became evident. First, holding Andy back a year to let his speech catch up a bit was not an option. He was extremely tall for his age and was already taller than all of the kids in his age range. Holding him back a year would only serve to make him stand out even more. Perhaps more importantly, Andy was more than ready to be challenged intellectually. He was ready to learn and holding him back would not be the best thing for him in the long run. The AIU sponsored a speech-language kindergarten with a very small class size. Each child in the class was supposed to have a primary diagnosis of a speech and/or language disorder. The class was taught by a speech-language pathologist. Speech therapy, occupational therapy, and physical therapy were all available right in the building and would be built into Andy's schedule. The kids from the speech-language classroom would also be integrated into the school's typical kindergarten class for art and gym and whatever else possible. Best of all, our school district just happened to host the program. Andy would be getting the therapy he needed, in the amount that he needed it, and he would be following the curriculum of his home school district. I had found the perfect placement for Andy!

Everything seemed to be going along okay as the school year started. Then came the first field trip and Andy was so excited to be going to visit the farm. And I was excited to be chaperoning my son's first field trip. I had always volunteered to chaperone Kate's field trips and really enjoyed the experiences. Kate always thought it was fun to have me along, so I was looking forward to doing the same for Andy. The day arrived and it was a perfect fall day in western Pennsylvania, cool, crisp, and sunny. I walked Andy to the classroom to let him get settled with his classmates. The teacher and the mothers from the typical kindergarten class were also standing around the door waiting for the kids to get in a line. I noticed that the other mothers were kind of looking at me strangely, as if I shouldn't be there. Was I invading their space? Was there some special kindergarten ritual handshake I didn't know about? Whatever, I just wanted to be there for Andy and his friends anyway.

Soon enough the kindergarten teacher from the typical room came striding over to me and said, "Why are you here? You can leave now." Whoa, this was weird and uncomfortable.

"I'm the chaperone for the speech-language classroom," I said perhaps a little too brightly.

"You don't belong here," the kindergarten teacher spat back at me. "There is no room on the bus for the special needs mothers!" Wow, in all my years of raising children with special needs no one had ever spoken to me like that. I could feel my face burning red. I saw Andy looking right at me. I couldn't even yell at her!

"Well," I said, "I'll just follow along in my car and join up at the farm."

"That's not necessary," the teacher shrieked. "You can just go home. We have it covered." *Oh please don't let me start to cry now*, I thought. I bent down to Andy and asked if he would be okay if I didn't go. He was so excited to be riding the bus, he didn't really care where I was and that was a good thing. I still don't know what the right thing was to have done. I could have really made a huge scene, but how would Andy have perceived that? Truly, I don't think it made any difference to him if I was there or not, but just slinking away has left a bitter taste in my mouth when I think about it.

It was just a month or so later that I had my second run in with the same kindergarten teacher. It was Thanksgiving and the kids had been working on a pageant for the parents: American Indians, Pilgrims, and turkeys, the whole shebang. The typical class and speech-language class had been combined for the show and we parents all stuffed ourselves into the kindergarten room that the mainstreamed kids used for class. All eyes were fixed on the kindergarten teacher as she stood to make her introductions. It went something like this, "Could all the children from the speech and language class please stand up? These are the special education students and they are not regularly in our class." I didn't actually hear much after that. What I learned that day was that you could actually be angry enough to see red. Again I ask, what the heck are you supposed to do? You're just so limited with all those little eyes watching you. The "perfect" placement for Andy I had fought so hard for had turned into a nightmare even I couldn't have imagined. I did nothing. I sat quietly with a frozen smile pasted in my face and watched the pageant and watched Andy say the line that months before he would not have been able to utter. Later on I ranted and raved about that kindergarten teacher to whoever would listen, but right then, I did nothing.

All that said, I would probably do it again given the choice. The hurt and pain that teacher caused was mine and mine alone. Andy was just fine, really more than fine. He had more therapy in that school year than I could have ever provided for him on my own. The speech-language classroom was a kindergarten through-first-grade program. Andy sat on the kindergarten side and did the first grade curriculum. Clearly he was ready to move on and that was what he wanted. His number one goal through that entire year was to get into the same school as his sister and that was what he accomplished in the speech-language kindergarten. The next year Andy was welcomed to Lincoln Elementary with open arms where he attended first grade in his home school, with his sister.

(kate)
It's all about spell check

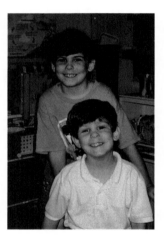

It seems to be universally understood these days that children with disabilities are far more likely to be bullied in school than other children. I was lucky, I was never really bullied in elementary school. When I was pulled out of class to see the speech therapist, none of the other kids seemed to notice or care. Lots of kids are pulled out of class in elementary school for lots of different reasons and no one ever even asked where I went. It was never a big deal to me because I really enjoyed spending time with my speech therapist. My speech therapist in grade school had to have had the most difficult name to pronounce for a kid with apraxia: Mrs. Lazarchick. Oh, the irony!

Mrs. Lazarchik was fun and I looked forward to the time I spent with her. Sometimes I had a joint session with some of the other kids who saw her for speech and I especially looked forward to those days, too. We played games and that was always more fun than what was going on in the classroom.

I was pulled out of my classroom for speech therapy from kindergarten through third grade. After seven long and tedious years of speech therapy, I was dismissed in third grade and forever freed from speech therapy, or at least that's what I thought at the time. Two years later, in fifth grade, I was once again pulled out from class. I was having difficulty with some of the words in science and geography. I kept a list of the words that gave me a hard time, and once a month I met with Mrs. Lazarchik and we went over each word individually until I had the motor plan; then I practiced the word on my own until I had it down.

Unlike those earlier years of speech therapy, I absolutely hated these sessions. Not only was I older, but I just didn't like getting pulled out of class as much as I had when I was seven. At eleven, you're just want to "fit in," and "be cool," and most importantly, be like everyone else. Getting pulled out of class made me different, and at eleven that was the worst thing imaginable.

I think I was lucky that most of my speech therapy came when I was younger. I am certain that I would have hated speech therapy as much as Andy did if I would have had to go as long as he did. Andy went to speech therapy through the eighth grade, at which point he decided he was done. I'm not sure how happy Mom was with that, but Andy was adamant and so he was done.

Although I "graduated" from speech therapy when I was in third grade, apraxia was still there lurking in the background. It was always there just under the surface and Latin seemed to bring out the worst in me and my apraxia. After I left elementary school and moved up to middle school, I started taking Latin to fulfill the middle school language requirement. All students took Latin in seventh grade. In eighth grade students could continue with Latin or switch to Spanish or French. My mom I and decided that staying with Latin for two years was probably the best bet. We had this theory that because Latin was a "dead" language and not really spoken anywhere, it might be a good fit for a kid with apraxia.

I'd like to think of myself as someone who doesn't give up when things become difficult, but from almost the first week I started with Latin, it became my worst nightmare. I'm not entirely sure how someone without apraxia learns a foreign language, but I know for a fact that it takes a heck of a lot more effort for a person with apraxia to learn one. For me, it became a memorization game.

From the moment I started learning Latin it was all about memorization. I was forced to memorize word meanings, spellings, and an entirely new grammar system, along with the history of Latin. Despite the fact it was a dead language, we were still required to read out loud, which added pronunciation to the list of things that kept me up at night with respect to Latin. This language was not dead. It was a living, breathing nightmare!

Spelling was something else that always gave me trouble in school. If my spelling in English was horrible, my spelling in Latin was abominable. My misspellings were the difference between a past tense verb and a present tense verb and the difference between a passing grade and failing.

At first, I did not make the connection between my difficulty with the foreign languages and my apraxia. The reality was that I learned English differently than most kids, so it would stand to reason that I would have to learn a foreign language differently also. Learning a foreign language is probably not impossible for kids with apraxia, but I do think it would have to be taught a lot differently for us.

On a Latin test, misspelling a word was the difference between the correct tense and a wrong answer. I spell words the way I pronounce them which is not always correct. My strategy was to just memorize everything. There is only so much memorization the teenage brain could do and as a result, my Latin grades were not stellar.

We were never lucky enough to find that teacher who could understand the issue and then adapt the curriculum. Instead, my teachers assumed I was not working hard enough or maybe just not smart enough.

In the end, I took Latin for five years and fulfilled the middle school and high school requirements. Fortunately for Andy, my mom was able to have his high school language requirement waived, and then we were able to have my college waive their language requirement. Finally, I felt like a huge burden had been lifted from my back. At least in Calculus 2 they spoke English!

Beyond Latin, apraxia reared its ugly head here and there in high school. Whenever I had to read something out loud I would stumble on the words, but it wasn't anything anyone would really notice. The worst part of reading out loud though is that after reading a couple sentences my mouth would get tired and my words would start to slur a little. This also happens to me when I'm not feeling well. The best way I can explain it is that sometimes my entire mouth becomes so heavy that I am suddenly aware of every single movement of the muscles in my mouth.

Because of my struggles with new words, I am not adventurous with my vocabulary. I don't use a wide assortment of vocabulary words in my expressive language in everyday life. I grew up knowing that I would not be able to pronounce certain words or unfamiliar words, so instead of embarrassing myself, I only use the words I am sure I know. There was a distinct difference between my in-class essays and the essays I was able to work on at home. Anytime I had to write something in class, I would stick to the words that I knew how to spell. At home I could be more experimental and use spell check.

Now that I've graduated college, I suspect apraxia may continue to affect my life and the choices that I make. I love to create characters and situations and it is my hope to be able to continue to do that as a professional. Apraxia continues to influence the way that I write. However, if having to depend on spell check and the thesaurus are the two biggest lasting effects of having apraxia, I think I'm going to be just fine growing up in the entertainment industry.

(kathy)

What about the bullies?

It was not a call I wasn't expecting, but when it came I was shocked, devastated, and just plain angry. There was only one week of school left and I thought we had made it through and my son was safe. But he wasn't. From second grade on, my son had been tortured by 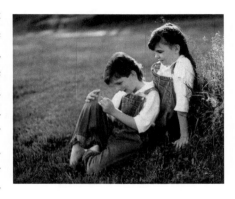 first one group of children and then another. By fourth grade, the first group had moved on to some other hapless child, but Andy was still having nightmares about them. He would wake up convinced that they were at his second-story window, staring at him as he slept.

The school was definitely proactive on the issue of bullying and they did what they could to keep things under control, but not every hallway and bathroom can be monitored every single minute of the school day. The principal and counselor focused on educating the children and raising their awareness and sensitivity levels.

All the same, by fourth grade, ten-year-old Andy was the target of children who, for whatever reason, felt better about themselves after making Andy feel humiliated. Andy and I had dealt with this all year. The counselor and I worked with Andy to give him strategies to cope with these children. He knew there were people in the building who supported him and that he could go to them if he needed help. When push came to shove, though, he employed none of those strategies and sought out no adult to help him.

Andy's class was in the art room and because it was the end of the school year and clean-up time, there was a lot of unstructured activity in the class. One of the boys that had been at the center of much of Andy's torment asked Andy to sit down next to him. I feel like what happened next was largely my fault. I raised my son to be kind and to always hope for and expect the best from other people. And that was exactly what he was doing when he sat down next to that child. Later, Andy told me he thought that this kid finally wanted to be friends with him. Andy sat down. Andy sat down on the tacks that the child had placed on the chair. I am not sure what happened next. What I do know is that Andy did not tell the art teacher. Finally, because he was in pain and humiliated, he told his classroom teacher. She sent Andy to the school nurse and the nurse called me.

Because I was PTA president, I was always in the office and around the school anyway. I'm not sure that my rushing to the school and flying into the office actually had any impact. When I got to the school Andy was traumatized and in tears. I called our pediatrician to make sure that Andy was up-to-date on his tetanus shots and then I did the thing that still makes me feel like the worst parent that has walked the planet: I sent him back into that classroom. I knew he had to go back and face his bullies. If he didn't, he would look back on the incident with shame. Andy knew that every child in that class knew what had happened. But he and I both were surprised at the support he found when he went back to the classroom. Later that evening, my phone started to ring as children went home and told their parents what had happened. The other children in Andy's class were so upset that he had been violated in that manner. It seemed like even though they may not want to be his best friend, it upset them to see him hurt and embarrassed.

So whatever happened to the child who hurt Andy? It became very important to me that the other children in that school see that treating someone with disrespect would not be tolerated. I insisted that this child be held accountable. I entrusted my son to their care and now it was time for the school to step up to the plate. The child received an in-school suspension and spent the remaining week of school outside of his regular classroom. Do I think this made him see the light and change his ways? No, indeed just the opposite, I think it inflamed him and made him angrier, but he thought twice before approaching Andy.

The problem here was not that the school didn't recognize this child as troubled. They did. It wasn't that no one tried to help him. They did. The problem from where I sat was that this child's parents refused to see their son for what he had become: a bully. And they refused to do anything to help him or to let the school help this child. Without the support of the parents, I don't believe there is any bullying program in the world that will be effective. As long as this is the case, children like Andy remain at risk at the hands of children who, for whatever reason, are bullies.

The saddest part of the whole story happened later when I began to teach Andy that there were some people in the world who just were not nice. I had to teach him that as kind as he might be to someone, they may still only want to hurt him. I taught him that trust is a gift that not everyone deserves. I taught him that sometimes his openness might lead to what we eventually named, "the great tack attack" and that perhaps he should hold back just a little. But most importantly I had to teach my son that even though there may be children who hurt him, he was smart and funny and a wonderful human being and that he had to have enough strength and faith to believe that and never, ever change.

(kate)

He's my brother and my hero

Having a child diagnosed with apraxia is rare enough, but having two children diagnosed with that particular speech disorder is pretty much unheard of, unless you're a Hennessy. Although I'm two and a half

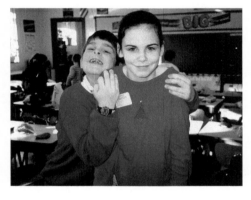

years older than Andy, he was diagnosed with apraxia first. His symptoms at age three were so much more severe and textbook that it was obvious to his speech therapist what was going on with him. I was five, and although I had already been in speech therapy for more than two years, my therapist decided to reevaluate my speech with apraxia in mind. I had previously been diagnosed as developmentally delayed, but as it turned out, I would also wear the diagnosis of apraxia. My treatment was modified for my diagnosis.

When I think about it, I wonder how my mother stayed sane. It was like we lived in the apraxia house. To a large extent, our lives really did revolve around our diagnoses. Andy and I were lucky to have each other growing up. From the very beginning, I knew there was someone else who struggled. I always knew another child who, like me, had problems talking. Neither Andy nor I ever worried about being different because in our house, apraxia was normal.

My mom says that when we were younger, I always understood what Andy was trying to say. In fact, according to her, I was Andy's interpreter. Having a sibling with a disability wasn't always easy though, as I'm sure it wasn't always easy for Andy. After a while it was difficult for anyone to tell that I even had apraxia. Andy was not so lucky. In addition to speech apraxia, he lived with a multitude of other diagnoses, one of which was sensory integration disorder that kept him off balance a lot, falling down and bumping into people. Andy never had a great perception of where he was in relation to other things in the world.

When I was a kid, we went to Disneyland in California a couple of times a year. The flight out could get pretty interesting with a kid who didn't have great control over his limbs. I remember one flight in particular when Andy kept accidently bumping the seat in front of him because he just didn't understand how close it was to him. My mom kept attempting to apologize to the woman and explain his issues to her. No matter how many times my mom tried to help Andy stay still, it just wasn't going to work. That woman was having none of it. She was not even willing to try to understand what was happening to the little kid sitting behind her. Wherever she is in the world today, her meanness is what I remember about her.

Once we got to Disneyland and had to stand in line for the rides, my mom positioned Andy in the middle of us so that he would bump into her or me and not some random stranger. Andy had very little control over his body, but other people thought he was just clumsy. I know as a child I never truly grasped just how entirely out of control his body was for him.

Andy's life in elementary school was torture for him. He was bullied in ways that I will truly never understand. It breaks my heart that Andy had to go through the things that he did and I will never be able to understand how kids can be so malicious.

It wasn't until high school that I began to feel responsible for Andy and become his advocate. When I was younger I just didn't get it. But by my senior year in high school I did. It was one of those beautiful May afternoons that you wait for all winter and quickly find your shorts when it finally arrives. Everyone was outside on the quad, throwing Frisbees, playing hacky sack, and just loving being outside. I was making my way down to the athletic field with some friends when I heard some shouting. I turned to see where the sound was coming from and I saw Andy in the middle of a group of guys. At first, I thought they were throwing a Frisbee around and I was excited to see Andy having fun. Then I realized that what they were throwing was my brother's fancy calculator in a mean-spirited game of keep-away. Hadn't he already been through enough? Couldn't they just let him do his math homework in peace? Clearly not! I was paralyzed for a minute, Andy was a sophomore in high school and I didn't want to embarrass him by coming to his rescue, but at the same time I wasn't about to let the jerks pick on my brother. It took just a second for me to decide I needed to get involved.

I threw down my bag and marched right up to the bullies. I began to shout at them. I was a senior and a girl, so clearly I had the advantage. They laughingly tried to make it seem like it was all in fun and Andy was part of it. I didn't buy it for one second. I put my face in the pack leader's face and yelled some more. I finished by informing him that if he didn't give Andy his calculator back I was heading straight to the headmaster's office and letting him know how they had all been smoking joints behind the boy's dorm. The stupid sophomore freaked out, gave Andy his calculator, and ran away with his tail between his legs.

What made me so furious about that afternoon was that I was not the only one who saw those boys giving my brother a hard time. Literally, a hundred students had walked past them and not one single person had done a thing. I will never understand that. It was so easy to stop it. Why was I the only one who tried?

It matters and it does make a difference. It made a difference to Andy and he carries his pain like a badge of honor. Those boys who tormented Andy in grade school and middle school probably never even think about Andy, but Andy carries the pain they caused every day of his life.

The seventy million Americans born during the eighties and nineties are known as Generation Y, the generation of children who grew up with technology and 97% of us own a computer, 94% a phone, and 76% of us use Instant Messaging. In spite of the innovation occurring in the world around us, bullying seems to be something we just can't or won't do anything about.

Walk down the hallway of any high school in America and the most common words heard are "test," "studying," "lunch'" and "retarded." The words 'retard' has become an everyday word for the kids of Generation Y. Most people hear that word and don't think twice about it. So what's the big deal about using the word "retarded" anyway? Everyone does it. After all aren't people who are different strange and scary?

People with disabilities, including Andy and me, have worked really hard to do what comes easily and naturally to others.

Using derogatory words takes away from all our hard work. The word "retard" is just like any racial or homophobic slur. The only difference is that people with cognitive disabilities often cannot stand up for themselves. Children who cannot communicate effectively don't have the resources to defend themselves, nor do they have the ability to tell anyone what is happening to them. But we all have feelings. Generation Y needs to make the choice to be the generation that cares about all of the people who are part of our community. Generation Y needs to be the generation that cares about the words they use.

I know that while growing up, I certainly wasn't the best sister I could have been to Andy. I was too worried about fitting in with everyone and being cool. I thought it was hard sometimes to have a sibling that was not like every single other person. I was wrong. Andy should be singled out and held up as the role model. Andy should be proud of who he was, who he is, and who he will become.

Today, Andy most certainly still deals with the effects of all the bullying he had to endure as a kid. He wears sarcasm as his life vest and tries hard to be grumbly. It's his way of keeping his heart safe. It makes me sad that he thinks he has to be this way. But to us, my mom and me, he is goofy and funny and really a big guy with a soft heart. But he's been hurt so many times that I worry that he doesn't know how to be vulnerable anymore.

I have watched as Andy has grown from the adorable, blonde, curly-haired little boy who loved Mario and Luigi to be a resilient and brave young man who still loves his fair share of video games. I will never be able to even imagine the pain that Andy has experienced at the hands of other children, but despite everything, he has triumphed and he has succeeded. I cannot wait to see where the road leads for him and I am so incredibly grateful to be able to have Andy as my brother. I am grateful to have him as my hero.

(kathy)
We are not alone,
we never were

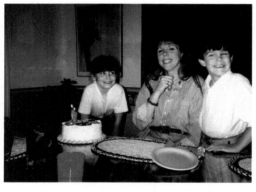

I'm not a comfortable flyer. I always wanted to think of myself as a great adventurer. One of those folks who could have her bags packed in ten minutes and with sparkling eyes be ready for anything. The fact is, I've never left my children and I've never been that upset about it. To me, a fabulous day is having everyone one at home looking for adventure in our own neighborhood. But in 2002, the CASANA Board of Directors began to plan the first Research Symposium on childhood apraxia of speech in Scottsdale, Arizona and I knew I would want to be there. But let's start at the beginning...

Sharon Gretz and Dave Hammer, M.A., CCC-SLP put together a workshop in the mid-1990s. By the time I got the flyer, I was a few years into dealing with apraxia and I had never met another parent who had children like mine. I had always felt like I was fighting this battle on my own. I quickly sent in my registration but I was too late, the workshop was already filled and that was that. Then they decided to do a second presentation because there was such an overwhelming response from people wanting to attend. The people who met one another at that workshop formed the Apraxia Parent Group in Pittsburgh. We met once a month and shared our stories, our setbacks, our victories, and the lessons we had learned. After those meetings, some of us would hang around and talk about our dreams. We often talked about our children and wondered how it would all turn out, but we also dreamed bigger dreams.

I clearly remember when the seed was planted for the *Time to Sing* CD late one night in a parking lot. We were talking about how hard it was for our kids to sing the songs all the kids sang in preschool sitting in circle time. Our kids felt left out and sad. We talked about how wonderful it would be if we could slow it all down and give our kids a chance to sing. Bob Moir and Mary Sturm took the "what if" and made it happen in 2000 when *Time to Sing* was released.

The research symposium started in much the same way. What if we could bring all the people who cared about apraxia, who cared about our children, together in the same room? "Can you even imagine what that would be like," we wondered? That idea began to hatch around the same time as the CD and in much the same way. Lots of things happened over the years, personally and professionally, and we all still had children that needed lots of attention, but we always came back to the idea of a research symposium.

The Childhood Apraxia of Speech Association of North America (CASANA) officially came into existence in the year 2000, and the Research Symposium became a reality in 2002. One of the things that became very important to the Board of Directors of CASANA was that families had to be represented at this Symposium. We really wanted the researchers to understand that not only were we trying to support them in every way possible, but that our children were the faces of apraxia.

After September 11, 2001 there were two things I said I never wanted to do: one was to get on a plane and the other was to leave my family. But early on the morning of February 28, 2004, I did just that, and with Mary Sturm, CASANA Board President, by my side, I left my children more than well cared for, got on a plane, and flew to Scottsdale, Arizona. I never really knew that palm trees and cactus grew side-by-side.

My stomach was very jittery, even after I got off the plane. I was not entirely sure I was really up for this "scientific" symposium. I have a degree from a very wonderful women's college in the Midwest, I create inclusive programming for children of all abilities, and I can keep the official score at a basketball game, for heaven's sake! But I was about to enter the world of people I idolized, people whose books I read and careers I followed, people who had gotten me through some of the most difficult moments of my life. Not only was I about to meet these folks, but I was going to represent parents of children with apraxia and participate in the Research Symposium! Turn the car around-I'm not ready!

When we first arrived, Mary and I found Sharon Gretz and Carol Myers setting things up for the next day. This was the first time I would meet Carol from the Hendrix Foundation, although we had talked on the phone and through e-mail a bit. The first night was amazing! It started with everyone gathering for a kind of get-to-know-you reception. The food was fabulous. I chatted with the Pittsburgh people I knew, Dave Hammer, M.A., CCC-SLP, Tom Campbell, Ph.D., CCC-SLP, and Chris Dollaghan, Ph.D., CCC-SLP. I met Larry Shriberg, Ph.D., CCC-SLP, Michael Crary, Ph.D., CCC-SLP, Shelly Velleman, Ph.D., CCC-SLP, and Edy Strand, Ph.D., CCC-SLP. They were all wonderful and personable and just regular people who cared about our children a whole lot. My eyes were constantly drawn to the pictures of the children that surrounded the perimeter of the room. The pictures were of children with apraxia, sent in by their parents, with messages to the researchers. I kept noticing that the researchers were as captivated and charmed by them as I was. One by one, they made their way around the room, as if to introduce themselves to the little ones whose voices they were fighting to find.

That first night was a kaleidoscope of new names and faces, but the evening ended with the folks from the CASANA Board, and a couple of the researchers just chatting around the fire pit late into the night.

By 8:00 a.m. the next morning, we were off and running. The researchers sat around long tables arranged in a big "U" shape, those of us who had been invited as guests sat at tables arranged in an "L" shape on the outside of the researchers. We had enough paper and pencils and little mints to get us through the day! I will leave it to others, who can do a better job than I can, to tell you what was said over the course of the Symposium, but I was mesmerized. Honestly, some of the material on brain function was a bit hard to follow, but I will say that most of the information was fairly palatable to the lay person.

There was one person who I had been very anxious to hear speak and that was Farenah Vargha-Khadem, Ph.D. Dr. Vargha-Khadem is the Head of the Department of Developmental Cognitive Neuroscience at the Institute of Child Health, University College, London and Head of the Unit of Clinical Neuropsychology at Great Ormond Street Hospital for Children. She had recently been investigating genetic issues and speech-language disorders. It goes without saying that with two children affected by apraxia, she is someone worth watching. As she spoke, I came to realize that she cares very deeply for the KE family, an extended family being studied by experts about half of whom, over three generations, have a confirmed diagnosis of childhood apraxia of speech, and she treats them with enormous respect and dignity. They are more than just a research tool for her; and she is fiercely protective of them. After her talk, we spoke briefly, but I was a little intimidated.

In the middle of the desert, for two days we focused on apraxia. It was a very humbling experience to hear the discussions that went on, to see the respect these folks have for one another, and to witness their willingness to argue a point and then learn from each other. I believe that our children are in good hands. At night, in our hotel room, Mary and I were like two teenagers at a slumber party. We stayed up late into the nights reviewing everything that had been talked about during the day.

The last night in Scottsdale, we had a very festive dinner to close the whole event. I was very excited when Dr. Khadem sat down at the table with Mary and me. She talked about her work and where she thinks the research is headed and how it will all turn out. She asked me about my children and then listened carefully as I talked about the struggles of having two children with apraxia. We talked a lot about the differences in their recoveries. She listened to my thoughts on apraxia and never once made me feel like I was "just a mom." I think she is exactly what my mother was talking about when she talked about being a "lady." I hope we meet again.

Soon enough, it was time for Mary and me to leave to catch the red-eye home. We both wanted to be home when our kids woke up in the morning. I found it impossible to sleep on the flight. I had 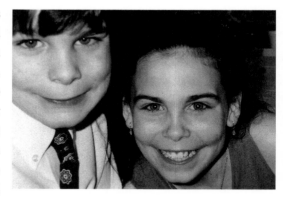 faced my fear, gotten on a plane, and met some of the people who had had the most impact on the lives of my children. How often does that happen? Of all the things I learned that weekend, perhaps the most important was that there are people out there working very hard for our children. We are not alone, we never were.

(kate)
The research study

In 2007, I took part in a study organized by Kathy Jakielski, Ph.D., CCC-SLP and one of her students, Ms. Melanie Green from Augustana College. We were in Anaheim, 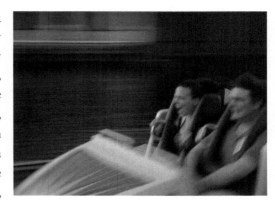 California at Disneyland for the Childhood Apraxia of Speech Association's National Conference. Dr. Jakielski and Melanie set up the study in one of the empty conference rooms and we got started right after the conference wrapped up.

At Dr. Jakielski's presentation at the 2008 Annual Convention of the American-Speech-Language-Hearing she explained the study this way:

"Given the severe nature of CAS, even when a child's speech impairment has resolved to normalcy, one might suspect that residual motor speech programming difficulty could exist sub-clinically. This difficulty could be evidenced at times when the

individual is under stress and/or fatigue. In this pilot study, we investigated whether or not an adolescent with an early history of CAS (KA) who now presents with normal speech continued to show the effects of CAS when undergoing challenging speech production tasks. Two other adolescents, one with a history of non-CAS speech impairment (ES) and the other with no history of speech impairment (CN), underwent the same challenging speech production tasks for purposes of comparison.

Research Questions

1. When completing challenging speech tasks (i.e., temporally- and phonetically-difficult speech productions), what is the performance of the three participants?

2. How does the performance of each participant compare with the performance of each of the other participants?

3. Are there unique speech characteristics of the participant who had a history of CAS, and if so, what are those characteristics?"

At the time, I wasn't thinking much about the design of the study or what the outcomes could mean in the field of childhood apraxia of speech. My part in the study didn't take very long at all, but participating in that study changed everything.

After going to speech therapy for seven years, sometimes five days a week, I "graduated" when I was in the third grade. By the time Dr. Jakielski approached me about participating in the study, I had been considered "resolved" for over eight years. With strategies in place, I did not really think much at all about my speech. I wasn't worried at all about helping Dr. Jakielski out with her research and what it might mean to me personally. Plus it was an excuse to hang out with Kathy J.

I do remember thinking that the whole thing might be a little boring if we were going to be doing the same kinds of things that I used to do in speech therapy: repetition, repetition and then more repetition. But I figured I could get this done and still have time to sneak away into Disneyland with Andy. I could not have been more wrong.

I knew going into the study that the whole point was to see if the researchers could "break down" my speech. I honestly believed that because I was resolved, it would be an impossible task: my speech was fine. I knew the apraxia was still there, somewhere, because I still made some mistakes in my speech now and then. But never did I imagine that Dr. Jakielski would be able to make me sound the way that I did back when I was in speech therapy, and I really never anticipated it would be quite so easy for her to do so. What I didn't know going into this study was that I was just about to find out how close to the surface my apraxia really was.

I felt so many emotions in that short hour. That hour that took forever. Even though I believed that I had come to appreciate what it meant to have apraxia, I hadn't been to speech therapy in over eight years. It's one thing to talk about apraxia when you know that you have apraxia, but no one else is able to tell anymore. It's easy to talk about apraxia when you don't sound like you have apraxia, and when you've crossed to the other side of the street and you're looking back over your shoulder. It's a whole different experience when the object of the game is to get you to make those mistakes again. It's difficult when the only way to discover what resolved apraxia really means is to try and discover what mistakes lay right under the surface.

Imagine my surprise in the little conference room with Dr. Jakielski and Melanie Green, when I couldn't perform the simple tasks put in front of me. Again and again, I failed. I was so ashamed. There I was a sixteen-year-old, soon to be junior in high school, and my mouth just would not go where I wanted it to go. I could not believe this was happening to me. Everything everyone had ever explained about apraxia was 100% true! The idea that your brain is somehow disconnected from your mouth was heartbreakingly true. I had strategies. This was not supposed to happen. I had therapy! I was resolved!

I remember becoming so frustrated that I couldn't get my mouth to work right. I was so embarrassed and I felt like I wasn't very good at talking. I felt as if the past eight years had never happened and that I was all of a sudden back in kindergarten and not able to talk. I had forgotten what that felt like. It felt like failure.

For most of the hour I was on the brink of tears. The experience was heartbreaking and eye-opening. I wasn't sure what they would discover when Kathy J. and Melanie began to calculate the results of the study, but what I learned that day was that although it can be resolved, apraxia never truly goes away.

Participating in this study was really important for me. It put much of my life in perspective, it gave me renewed appreciation on how much work it is for the little ones with CAS to learn to talk. It had been so long since I had been up close and personal with my apraxia that I had even begun to doubt that my diagnosis had been correct. No question there anymore! People who know me now and didn't know me when I was younger find it hard to believe there was a time that speaking was difficult for me. It's hard for them to imagine a time when I didn't sound like I do now. But this study reminded me of the battle that I fought and the battle that I won. It reminded me of all the work that I put in to my speech before I even knew what that meant. It also reminded me of all the work that goes into my speech every day of my life, even though I don't always realize it.

So what does it really mean to have resolved apraxia? In my humble, non-professional opinion, I think that resolved apraxia means something different for everyone. For me, it means that after seven years of speech therapy I can walk up to people on the street and they can understand what I'm saying. It means I don't have to spend countless hours in speech therapy and it means that I can go about my everyday life and not have to even think about apraxia all the time. That being said, apraxia undeniably still affects my everyday life. I still have trouble pronouncing certain words, and whenever I'm really tired, talking in general is definitely much more difficult. It's during these times that I can almost feel every muscle in my mouth and forming words is just hard.

Here's what the Dr. Jakielski and Melanie Green concluded regarding that study; *"KA produced the highest number of errors, the largest variety of errors, and errors on more subtests than the other two participants. Although both ES and KA had complete phonetic inventories and no evidence or reports of speech deficits in adolescence, including at the time of testing, their performance on the experimental tasks revealed continued difficulty producing speech requiring complex temporal and phonetic productions.*

On many of the speech tasks, KA exhibited errors characteristic of CAS. Thoonen, Maassen, Gabreels, and Schreuder (1999) reported that performance on diadochokinesis could be used to distinguish CAS from other disorders of speech, and KA exhibited significant difficulty completing these tasks. KA also exhibited unusual consonant substitutions, as well as numerous vowel errors.

Given the very small sample size of this pilot study, these results cannot be extrapolated to other children with a history of speech impairment. A larger study currently is underway."

In the end, I am so glad I agreed to participate in the study with Dr. Jakielski and Melanie Green. It was eye-opening and humbling at the same time. In that moment, as I sat there in the little conference room in Disneyland, unable to perform the simplest of speech tasks, my connection with all the other children with CAS was crystallized. The one thing I did understand after that day was that no matter where I went or what I did in my life, I would be connected to all the kids with childhood apraxia of speech who would come after me.

(kathy)

Anything but silent

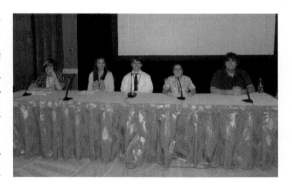

WooHoo! If you had asked me 18 years ago where we would be today, I could never have imagined our lives today. At CASANA's 2011 National Conference on Childhood Apraxia of Speech, I sat back in the audience of the last general session of the conference and watched my two children participate in the teen panel designed to answer the questions of parents who wanted to know what the future might hold for their young children and of therapists who never really get to see how the kids they treat turn out. It was the most amazing and humbling experience of my life, truly. My daughter was poised and thoughtful, and several times looked over at me and smiled while mentioning something I had done when they were kids. Kate has spoken at conferences all over the country and really is at ease in front of an audience. The conference was the first time that Andy spoke in front of any kind of audience. My gosh, the kid was hysterical and had the audience in the palm of his hand. Andy spoke honestly about the trials and tribulations of growing up with apraxia; at the same time, he radiated hope. To me, this was as good as it gets and in my wildest dreams I could never have imagined the scene that was in front of me.

Kate had been in therapy for seven years finishing up in the middle of third grade. Her only support came later in the form of a once-monthly meeting with her speech therapist to go over the list of words that gave her difficulty in the upper grades of elementary school. In 2004, Kate was asked to accompany me to Wilmington, Delaware to present a session on "How Apraxia Affects the Family." She did a great job and has been speaking regularly for the Childhood Apraxia of Speech Association since then.

Kate always loved sports and played basketball from grade school through high school. When she was junior in high school, Kate dislocated her knee cap and was out of sports for almost a year. During her recovery after knee surgery, Kate discovered film editing programs. When she wasn't in physical therapy rehabbing her knee, she was editing her favorite television heroine Buffy into another music video. Kate made it back to the basketball season in her senior year of high school, but then her other knee began to slide out of place and her doctor told her that a basketball career was pretty much over for her and she would not be able to play in college. Kate was going to have to find another outlet for her considerable energy. And it seemed like film could be just the thing.

When Kate was in high school the movie *Homecoming* was filmed at her school. Kate spent a couple hours on the phone and ended up with a job as a production assistant for a couple days on the set. Soon after that, she began work on *My Bloody Valentine, 3-D* as a production assistant and has worked on feature films steadily ever since.

Kate attends St. Mary's College in South Bend, Indiana, my alma mater, where she will graduate with a self-designed major in creative writing, and film with a minor in theater, and business administration.

Kate has a bright and shiny future ahead of her, a future that does not include a speech impairment. If you met Kate you would never suspect that she had any type of speech disability when she was a child. Although her initial prognosis was guarded, Kate has moved the mountains in her path and is finally exactly what she wanted to be-just like any other kid.

Kate is committed to reaching back behind her and giving a hand to the kids who are coming after her. She continues to advocate for children with apraxia as her schedule permits and I know that no matter where her future leads her, she will always support the kids who fight the battle she has already won. I am so proud of all that Kate has accomplished in her young life, but her commitment to being an advocate is what I am most proud of and what always makes me a bit weepy.

Where is Andy today? Remember the kid who was never going to speak at all? That kid is a sophomore at Case Western Reserve University majoring in electrical engineering. Not bad for a child who was never going to be able to function as a "normal" kid, right?

It was clear pretty early on that Andy was one smart kid. It always seemed like he got my jokes! I believe that it was Andy's intelligence that got him through the hard times. After twelve years of therapy Andy said, "No more!" When a kid reaches eighth grade you have to begin to respect his input and what he wants to do or not do. When kids are a little older, motivation is really one of the keys to success and he was not motivated to continue. Andy clearly understood there was a little more work that needed to be done on those pesky "r" sounds and a little bit of bilateral slushiness. Andy also clearly understands that if he wants to work on his residual speech errors, he can always go back and do so. For now though, he is done and I have to respect that.

Even though Andy has the heart of an engineer, he also has an artistic side. When he was in grade school he won awards for the music he wrote music on the computer. In high school Andy discovered theater. With my background being in theater, I couldn't have been more thrilled and we were able to work on several productions together.

But from the time he was a little boy, Andy loved computers. He was twelve years old when I handed over my computer to him and even now I do whatever Andy tells me to do with my computer. I was pretty sure that Andy would end up doing something with computers and I tried to do whatever I could to reinforce his interest. Andy attended computer camps and classes all through grade school, and then attended Andrew's Leap at Carnegie Mellon University and Governor's School at Drexel University.

Shortly before Andy graduated from high school, circumstances dictated that he become a man overnight. He stood by me through some really hard times, taking the lead in our lives when I needed him. And through it all, he maintained his ability to laugh and admire the absurd. He is at the same time sarcastic and terribly sweet. He walks to the beat of his own drum and is unafraid to be different. He is well liked by his peers, his teachers, and the people with whom he works. When he attends a CASANA conference, he is always greeted enthusiastically by the attendees, as well as by the speakers. Andy has become a person that I admire; he is the hero in the story of my life.

When my children were younger, I would cry in the shower because it was a safe place to really let out all my fears for their future. I couldn't even begin to imagine what the future would hold for these two little kids who had so many obstacles in their paths. My heart broke for them and fear was my constant companion. Today, I am humbled by their achievements, I celebrate 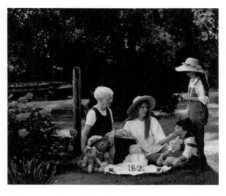 their journeys, and I am just so happy that God saw fit to put these two amazing and special children in my life.

(k a t e)

The epilogue, but not the end

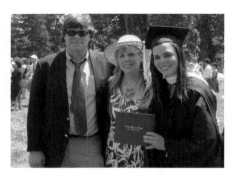

I started writing this book when I was fifteen and a sophomore in high school. I'm now finishing it as a twenty-two year old about to graduate from Saint Mary's College. It's crazy to think of how much has happened since then and how much has changed and, well, how much hasn't changed.

Andy and I have both been out of speech therapy for so long that it seems as if it were another lifetime ago. Just as my mother always made sure when we were growing up, apraxia does not define our lives. It does play a part, however.

In order to graduate from Saint Mary's, every senior must complete a senior comp project in their particular focus of studies. I am a self-designed, double major in creative writing and film and as a result, I was also able to design my senior comp. My senior comp was a full length screenplay for film. The next step was choosing a topic for the screenplay. I went back and forth and then settled back at apraxia. I wanted to write a screenplay about how my mom dealt with the discovery that her two small children struggled with a rare speech disorder known as childhood apraxia of speech. Writing a screenplay about my family and apraxia felt right. It fit.

The summer before my senior year of college I started to work on my screen-play, I had to create an outline and create depth to my characters. Once school began, I was in a class with other English Writing majors where we met once a week to review and critique our work. I was the only student writing a screenplay. As it turned out, I had to fight to keep my topic of apraxia. My professor could not seem to accept that one child could have such a devastating diagnosis, let alone two children in the same household. While I could see his point that it might be beneficial to keep the focus on one child with apraxia, I was dead-set on keeping it as authentic as possible. I would be the one who would do justice to my mother's story. I fought for my story. I wore the guy down, and finally he told me to start writing and "we'll see where it goes from there."

After about sixteen weeks of writing, I completed my comp and submitted it. There were so many times when I called my mom, upset about where the story was going or about one of my professor's critiques-so many times when I considered scrapping it because I didn't believe I was doing the best I could do. Just as my mom never gave up on Andy or me, I never gave up on her story. Even though I received an "A" for my work, the screen play is nowhere near really finished. I will keep working on it. My legacy will be our story.

So what now? Where do I go once I graduate?

I've been extremely lucky that I've known what I've wanted to do since I was a teenager, and even more lucky that I've been able to work in my field since I was a senior in high school. Once I graduate, I can finally work full-time and never have to turn down film work because I'm still in college. I absolutely love what I do! Hopefully I will be able to continue work on movies and television shows while I write. My dream is to direct and produce my own written work. If all that doesn't work out, I can become a reality show contestant!

The truth is, I've come a long way since my days in speech therapy, but in all honesty, I wouldn't change a thing. Apraxia is, and will forever be, part of who I am. Apraxia doesn't define me, but it is part of me. Those early years can be so difficult and heartbreaking, but if you can make it through the storm, everything that follows is so much sweeter.

I think struggling for something that comes so naturally for other people has helped to make my brother and me more aware of how lucky we really are. We learned resilience when we were just little kids and we know what it means to overcome the odds. As young adults, we are ready for whatever the future holds for us.

Volunteering for and attending so many of CASANA's conferences and workshops has also had an impact on me. I've met so many amazing and courageous parents, professionals, and volunteers over the years, each one inspiring me.

I have no idea what the future has in store for me, whether it be a career in the entertainment industry or something I've yet to discover, but I do know one thing for certain, wherever I end up, I will never forget my past, my childhood, or where I came from, to become the person I am today. At the end of the day, hope really does speak!

"Siyo nqoba"

One of the questions that I get asked the most regarding my childhood experiences with childhood apraxia of speech is "What do you remember?" My answer to that particular question is always the same: "Not much!" One thing I've learned is that children don't really remember anything much of anything. This observation has 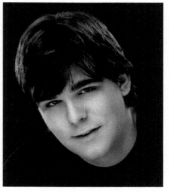 come after years of hearing my mother reminisce about childhood activities of which I have absolutely no recollection.

My earliest childhood memory is of preschool and wandering off into the woodlands surrounding the school and getting told not to do that again. Guess what? I did it again! But I do have a few hazy memories of those early years in speech therapy. I remember the waiting. I vividly remember the artificial tree in the lobby of the clinic. I also remember picking a leaf from that tree every time that we were in the waiting room. And every time I did my mother would gently remind me that the tree was not real and the leaf would not grow back. I guess my little brain couldn't comprehend a fake plant, so guess what I did? I picked more leaves. I have no idea how many times they replaced that plant. Which begs the question, "Why didn't they just put a real one in that waiting room?"

I was in and out of therapy from the earliest time that I can remember and continued until just about the end of my eighth grade year of school. By that point in my life I was sick of speech therapy. Skipping class had changed from being cool to annoying. I was attending a small private school in Pittsburgh, PA at the time. Private schools generally do not take federal money: they tend to use Individual Education Plans and 504's as toilet paper. The fact that I even had speech therapy in middle school is something to wonder about. At the time however, I didn't care; I just wanted to be like the other kids. I actually wanted to go to all of my classes! I know, I was a weird kid back then.

So, I told my mother that I was done with speech therapy. It was no longer worth anyone's time, effort, or monetary expense. I believe a reference to the Pareto Principle would not go unwelcome here. The effort it took to go from making my `r' sound ninety percent of the time to ninety-nine percent of the time was, quite frankly, not worth me falling behind in my academic classes anymore. To this day, I still have trouble pronouncing some speech and language constructs. There are words that I have absolutely no idea how to pronounce. Like my sister, when I am not at my mental peak, my speech begins to slur. But, during my day-to-day life, no one can tell that I was once diagnosed with a crippling speech disorder. At my university, exactly one person knows that I was even diagnosed with childhood apraxia of speech, and the only reason she knows is that she saw me editing a copy of this book during class and I had to explain to her what I was doing.

There are times when you look back on your life and say, "I chose this path and it changed the course of my life," One such moment occurred in December of my freshman year of high school. The previous month, one of my classmates had installed *Halo: Combat Evolved* on a hidden network share at school. Every day before school started we played the game. Our teams evolved into epic matches of "The Library Kids" vs. "The Rowe Hall Kids." Over winter break I copied the game to an ash drive to practice at home because, let's face it, a kid with motor planning issues and sensory integration disorder needs a little extra practice. I was always ranked last and I wanted to be better.

The problem with the trial edition of *Halo: Combat Evolved* was that it was limited to a single multiplayer map with two game types, which got very boring, very quickly. Working some Internet magic, I acquired a full copy of the game that did not need to be installed, and more importantly, had working multiplayer support. Over winter break I practiced on the "new" maps so that I could have a better ranking when school started again. (Remember: weird kid here.)

Loading the multiplayer server list, I selected the only server with people playing. It was the Gephyrophobia map that had quickly become one of my favorites. When I joined, there were three people playing on it. Two of them had the tag "/-GF]" in front of their name; the third person's name did not have a tag. The four of us played for what seemed like hours. Sometimes we gained a player or two, sometimes we lost a player who would quit after losing. Before I left the server for dinner, I typed the customary \ gg" (Good Game) into the chat window. Both of the players with tags commented on how they liked playing with me so much that they wanted me to join their "gaming clan." They gave me a web address to complete the application.

I thought long and hard about joining. I thought I was too young. I was under the mistaken impression that everyone on the series of tubes we call the Internet was a bad person, lurking in the shadows, ready to kidnap anyone stupid enough to join a forum or chatroom. It turns out that I have never been more wrong in my life. So, with eager anticipation, I submitted my application to join the Galactic Federation, a Star-Trek themed gaming clan specializing (at the time) in *Star Trek: Elite Force II and Halo: Combat Evolved.*

The day that I received the email congratulating me on being accepted, I was ecstatic. I had a clean slate. Absolutely no one knew who I was. I could be anyone that I wanted to be. Eventually I rose to be the Executive Officer of the entire clan, but at the moment I was a nervous new recruit. I read all of the information on the web forums, which instructed me to download and install two programs on my computer: Xfire and TeamSpeak. Xfire is more-or-less a chat program that can be used in-game. (It also has the added benefit of keeping track of how many hours one plays computer games.) The other program, TeamSpeak, also runs in the background, but instead of text messaging, it uses Voice over Internet Protocol (VoIP) to enable teammates to speak to each other. Using any kind of VoIP system is essential to being a well-organized team. The problem with any Voice over Internet Protocol system is, well, the voice part. The first time I joined the Teamspeak server I lied and said that my microphone was broken. I was incredibly nervous about these new friends I was in the process of making. Would they accept my slight speech problems? Would they even notice? As it turns out, they didn't notice. Not once in the three years I was actively in the clan did anyone make any comment about my speech.

That was one of the most confidence boosting things that ever happened to me. Random strangers who lived in Australia, Canada, and the United Kingdom could perfectly understand my rapid-fire instructions during games. *Counter-Strike*: Source games would last well into the night for me, playing against opponents all over this world, and each and every one of them could understand me.

And that brings me back to my title. One of the odd things that I do whenever I buy a new keyboard is to transcribe a movie. What seems like an unusual thing to do actually has several benefits, namely that at the end of two hours you are much more familiar with your new keyboard. Besides, who doesn't want an opportunity to re-watch an old favorite?

Several years back I had just received a new laptop and it was time to begin this ritual for the new device. This time, I chose the movie *The Lion King* to transcribe (mainly because I was too lazy to go downstairs and get a different movie, but minor details). As much as I love that movie, I had a horrible time making my script. That being said, at the end of the movie my touch typing on my new computer had improved tremendously. The trouble that I encountered was that some of the movie was not in English, but in the Zulu language. I have enough trouble spelling in English, let alone an obscure African language. I took the easy way out, which involved some Google magic with a little hint of Ctrl + C, Ctrl + V. My script was done, without me embarrassing myself over misspelled words. However, in my quest of not misspelling words that I had no clue how to spell in the first place, I came across a nugget of knowledge that had escaped me for years: the translations of the lines in the song *The Circle of Life*. Nestled between the lyric lines "Sithi uhhmm ingonyama" and "Ingonyama nengw' enamabala" (which translate to "Oh yes, it's a lion" and "A lion and leopard come to this open place", respectively), is the phrase "Siyo Nqoba," which translates to "We're going to conquer."

Ever since that night, that particular phrase has stayed with me. I remember back to my years of speech therapy, to the countless hours I spent out of the classroom, learning not math and grammar, but rather how to talk. I remember my struggles. At one point the professionals told my mother that I would never be able to talk, and it was a miracle I could even walk. I remember how I came out of all that being able to talk. I remember coming out on top after years of hard work. I remember that my mother, my sister, and I conquered childhood apraxia of speech.

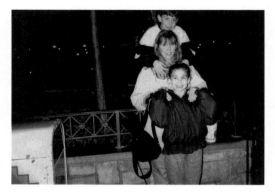